CW00858265

Aftershocks

Aftershocks

Politics and Trauma in Britain, 1918–1931

Susan Kingsley Kent
Professor of History, University of Colorado, Boulder, USA

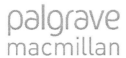

First published 2009 by
PALGRAVE MACMILLAN

Palgrave Macmillan in the UK is an imprint of Macmillan Publishers Limited,
registered in England, company number 785998, of Houndmills, Basingstoke,
Hampshire RG21 6XS.

Palgrave Macmillan in the US is a division of St Martin's Press LLC,
175 Fifth Avenue, New York, NY 10010.

Palgrave Macmillan is the global academic imprint of the above companies
and has companies and representatives throughout the world.

Palgrave® and Macmillan® are registered trademarks in the United States,
the United Kingdom, Europe and other countries.

ISBN-13: 978–1–4039–9333–5 hardback
ISBN-10: 1–4039–9333–5 hardback

This book is printed on paper suitable for recycling and made from fully
managed and sustained forest sources. Logging, pulping and manufacturing
processes are expected to conform to the environmental regulations of the
country of origin.

A catalogue record for this book is available from the British Library.

Library of Congress Cataloging-in-Publication Data
Kent, Susan Kingsley 1952 May 9–
    Aftershocks : politics and trauma in Britain, 1918–1931 / Susan
Kingsley Kent.
        p.   cm.
    Includes bibliographical references and index.
    ISBN-13: 978–1–4039–9333–5
    ISBN-10: 1–4039–9333–5
    1. Great Britain—Social conditions—20th century   2. Great
Britain—Politics and government—1910–1936.   3. War neuroses—Great
Britain—History—20th century.   4. World War, 1914–1918—Psychological
aspects—Great Britain.   5. World War, 1914–1918—Social
aspects—Great Britain.   I. Title.
DA578.K46 2009
941.083—dc22   2008035148

10   9   8   7   6   5   4   3   2   1
18   17   16   15   14   13   12   11   10   09

Printed and bound in Great Britain by
CPI Antony Rowe, Chippenham and Eastbourne

To all of those whose lives Elisa touched
and to
Anne, who has touched mine so profoundly

Contents

Acknowledgements   viii

Introduction   1

1   Britons' Shattered Psyche   10

2   Jews, "Blacks," and the Promises of Radical Conservatism,
    1919–1925   35

3   The Amritsar Massacre, 1919–1920   64

4   Reprisals in Ireland, 1919–1921   91

5   The General Strike of 1926   122

6   Flappers and the Igbo Women's War of 1929 (with Marc
    Matera)   149

Conclusion: Resolving the "National Crisis" of 1929–1931   180

Notes   196

Bibliography   218

Index   226

Acknowledgements

It has taken me 15 years to write this book. In that time I have incurred many, many debts, and I take great pleasure in being able now to thank everyone who helped me. Support from the Institute for Advanced Study, the National Endowment for the Humanities, and Phil DiStefano, Susan Avery, and Todd Gleeson at the University of Colorado gave me the time and space I needed to gather evidence, think, and write. At the Institute, I benefited from the intellectual and personal fellowship of Joan Scott, Ava Baron, Linda Gregerson, Stephen Mullaney, and Dan Sherman; the library staff there and at Princeton University provided me with untold riches. Jean Allman, Misty Bastian, Jeff Cox, Jim Cronin, Steve Feierman, Jane Gallop, Jane Garrity, Nicky Gullace, Holly Hanson, Janet Jacobs, Alison Jagger, Marc Matera, Marjorie McIntosh, Bob Moeller, Susan Pedersen, Lou Roberts, Sonya Rose, Diana Shull, Janet Watson, and Jay Winter offered opportunities, comments, criticisms, and suggestions that facilitated my research and writing. Thanks to you all.

At Palgrave, Michael Strang, Ruth Ireland, and Geetha Naren gave much-appreciated guidance, assistance, and support.

My good friends and colleagues Fred Anderson, Virginia Anderson, Carol Byerly, Phil Deloria, and Martha Hanna, and an unknown reader for a press that opted not to publish this book gave me incredibly helpful advice as I went about conceptualizing my arguments. They asked me to think much more carefully about the relationship between theory and practice and the book is the stronger for their contributions. I am most grateful to them. Jon Lawrence went through the manuscript with a keen eye for errors of fact and interpretation; his input and assistance strengthened the book immeasurably. I owe him big time. And my dear friend Bonnie Smith, who has talked with me about this book since its inception, gave generously of her time, energies, knowledge, and heart to ensure that it was as good as I could make it. I am deeply indebted to her.

The death of my niece, Elisa Kent Mendelsohn, in 1986 inspired me to investigate the issues of trauma and loss I treat in this book—I needed to know how people in the past handled such a terrible tragedy. This book is dedicated to her family, who feel the pain and the joy of her to this very day, and to Anne Davidson, who has been a constant source of love, laughter, and support.

Introduction

> To calculate the effect of mental and bodily suffering, not
> on a man but on a whole generation of men, may seem an
> impossible task.[1]

In the late fall of 1916, Ford Madox Ford, suffering from hallucinations
attributed to shell shock and noting the prevalence of men who displayed similar conditions, wondered "what the effect of it will be on us
all, after the war—& on national life and the like." His concerns anticipated the way the Great War would subsequently be conceptualized:
within months of the armistice, the war became portrayed not as a conflict between great powers, or even of men and materiél, but primarily
as a psychological event. As Valentine Wannop, a character in Ford's
Parade's End, put it in regard to her lover:

> the dreadful thing about the whole war was that...the suffering had
> been...mental rather than physical.... If he had been killed it would
> not have been so dreadful for him. But now he had come back with
> his obsessions and mental troubles.... Hitherto, she had thought of
> the War as physical suffering only; now she saw it only as mental
> torture...[and] the mental torture could not be expelled.

Veteran Charles Carrington, writing at the end of the 1920s, summed
up the war in a way that reflected the view prevailing by the early
years of the decade. "War is a contest of nerves," he declared. "That
army wins which in times of tribulation can longest bear the mental strain of plague, pestilence and famine; battle, murder and sudden
death." W.N. Maxwell, who served as chaplain to the 43rd Casualty
Clearing Station and the 6th Corps, wrote an account of the war in 1923

1

entitled *A Psychological Retrospective of the Great War*. Caroline Playne called her 1925 study of wartime *The Neuroses of the Nations*; her subsequent histories of the home front during the years 1914–1918, written in the 1930s, concerned themselves primarily with what she identified as the "most important" aspect of war time: "the psychology of social life, the state of men's minds under the influence of the stress and excitement of war... the prevailing mental fever and alienation from standards of sanity." In a 1924 novel, journalist Philip Gibbs described Britain as "a nation of neurotics," a state perhaps accounted for by Hilda Doolittle—HD—in her account of an air raid on London, in which her neighbor's house had been hit by a bomb and the windows of her own house blown out by the explosion. "What does that sort of shock do to the mind, the imagination," she asked a friend, "—not solely of myself, but of an epoch?"[2]

This question has occupied historians, critics, sociologists, and psychologists for decades now, and the attempts to answer it have yielded a rich cache of insights about the effects of industrialized warfare on the human psyche. In consequence, we know a great deal about what contemporaries called "shell shock," that unaccountable malaise of body and mind initially believed to be caused by the buffeting of exploding artillery shells, and in the belief that that knowledge holds good for all people across all time, have developed an entire diagnostic protocol for what we now term "post-traumatic stress disorder."[3] So pervasive has the concept of shell shock become in our understandings of the Great War that it not only serves as "a prism through which much of the cultural history of the 1914–1918 war has been viewed," as Jay Winter has put it, but has become a metaphor for the unprecedented nature—the size, scope, and consequences—of modern industrialized warfare.[4] The scholarship of shell shock has generated a large body of work on the culture of memorialization. Historians and literary critics have produced impressive accounts of the uses of memory to somehow accommodate the devastation of the Great War. Rituals of remembrance provided many sections of British society with relief from the traumas of war by turning back to earlier, traditional forms of expression for comfort or a sense of familiarity. Others retreated to the realm of the domestic, seeking peace and tranquility in the everyday activities of gardening, reading, and jig-saw puzzles.[5]

A second literature treats the political consequences of the war in "that extended war decade," as one historian has fittingly called it.[6] Detailed, insightful studies of colonial risings, feminism, and Labour,

Liberal, and Conservative politics abound, as do analyses of the relative strengths and weaknesses of British fascist organizations. Perhaps the most compelling question concerns the success of the Conservative party in maintaining its hold on the British voting public in the interwar decades. At a time when electoral reform had produced a new mass electorate of working-class and female voters, Conservatives managed to stay in power for all but three of the 20-odd years between the wars. They scored decisive wins in 1924, 1931, and 1935, but even when Labour won the premiership in 1923 and 1929 Conservatives had taken the majority of the popular vote. Attempts to explain this remarkable run have focused on a variety of factors—organization, management, leadership, ideology, discourse.[7] As one critic of this historiography has observed, these approaches have assumed more than they have illuminated; they have tended to treat voters as predictable members of sociological groups who needed merely to be mobilized by party organizers. He calls for studies analyzing the "discursive substance of Conservatism" to complement those of the institutional structures of the party.[8]

Surprisingly, the literatures of trauma and cultural memory on the one hand and of conventional politics on the other remain largely aloof from one another, though both refer to each other as a matter of course.[9] This book seeks to bring these two literatures together, to argue the crucial connection between structures of feeling and political culture in Britain and thereby to explain the widespread appeal of conservative politics to a broad segment of British public opinion. I want to extend Winter's insight to suggest that shell shock as a metaphor for the experience of the war turned into a new model of the mind, which, in turn, transmuted into a felt condition, an "experience," for millions of individual Britons. Individually as subjects and collectively as a society, Britons incorporated into their conscious and unconscious understandings of their political selves the meanings attached to the notion of shell shock, most particularly, the imagery that informed the view of the traumatized psyche as shattered. In countless and disparate accounts told during and after the war, men and women expressed their convictions that the traumas of war had torn them to pieces, fragmented their existences, utterly disrupting the flow of what should have been their natural lives.

The emotional and mental consequences of unbearable war-related experiences, enormous loss of life, and devastating grief for Britons that resulted in a new understanding of the shattered self played out on a national level, producing a particular set of policies and behaviors unlike those of an earlier time. The political force of emotions, to paraphrase one scholar[10]—particularly those associated with loss and mourning leading to post-traumatic stress disorder—must be appreciated if we are to truly grasp the political history of Great Britain in the first decade of the interwar period, a decade whose historians have generally failed to come to grips with the extraordinary violence—figurative if not always actual—visited upon those regarded as "un-English," whether they be immigrants from Europe, Jews, colonial subjects, or British citizens with suspect tendencies. Historians have usually identified the campaigns against these "others" with the so-called Die-Hards in parliament and their journalistic allies at the right-wing *Morning Post*, *National Review*, and *Spectator*, portraying them as an insignificant group of reactionary holdovers from the prewar years who would not accept the economic and political realities of democratic postwar society, out-lyers whose anachronistic attitudes and rearguard actions would doom them to the ashbin of Whiggish history. Conventional historiography paints the period as one dominated by moderate Conservatism, personified by the comforting and reassuring figure of Stanley Baldwin, a state arrived at by 1922 in part as a result of social integration achieved through annual acts of remembrance that purged "the demons of discontent and disorder" thrown up by the war.[11] Baldwin is given special prominence in this view of the period: one historian argues that he "tamed" democracy, largely through his oratory, by aligning it with constitutionalism and patriotism, incorporating what he regarded as the potentially dangerous "working masses of the people" in his vision of the whole of society. In order to "prevent the class war becoming a reality," as Baldwin put it, he transformed the public face of the Conservative party from one determined to snuff out socialism and promote the interests of the propertied to one that represented the whole nation. As this same scholar recognizes, however, Baldwin's message of a unified "Englishness" depended upon a contrast to "unEnglishness," qualities identified with what Baldwin called the "poisonous dogmas of foreign manufacture"—trade union militancy, general strikes, and socialism. The unity of the nation, in other words, could be established only by excluding those "exotic alien doctrines" that existed outside the nation as it was portrayed by Conservatism. However strident—even brutal— he might be in his depictions of "unEnglish" labor unionists or Labour leaders, Baldwin's favor with voters across the political spectrum never seemed to diminish,[12] a fact we ought to take heed of as we try to comprehend the remarkable popularity of interwar Conservatism. For the "demons of discontent and disorder" did not vanish after 1922, the attacks of the Die-Hards were not the lonely cry from the wilderness they have been thought to be. As Lord Salisbury wrote to Conservative party leader Andrew Bonar Law on 4 March 1922, the Die-Hards constituted "a genuine movement of honest men who have risked their political reputation in order if possible to rescue the Country, and however people may sneer such an effort always does good in the long run. And they are of course much more powerful in the country than they are in the House of Commons."[13] Indeed, a large proportion of Britons embraced the attitudes they represented and articulated them in a series of physical and linguistic assaults on "blacks," Jews, women, and workers throughout the 1920s. The forces of disorder—the threats to psychic wholeness—would not be vanquished until 1931, when the "crisis" facing the nation was resolved with the dismantling of the Labour government and the establishment of a National government in its place.

My thesis rests on at least three propositions. The first—that there is a relationship between "shell shock" and one's sense of self—and the second—that individual cases of trauma may be extrapolated to a larger entity, to a society, and that the individual subjectivity associated with trauma may be generalized to a nation to create a shell-shocked society—are treated in Chapter 1. I address the third proposition—that shell shock had a profound impact on national life, that shell-shocked Britain turned to certain political actions that sought to repair the collective psyche—in a series of chapters dealing with a variety of events and issues: the passage of the Aliens' Restriction Act of 1919, the race riots of 1919, and the response to France's introduction of black troops to Germany in 1920; the Amritsar massacre in 1919; the reprisals against the Irish in 1919–1921; the General Strike of 1926; and the debates over the bill to enfranchise women over 30 in 1927 and 1928 and the Igbo women's war of 1929. When collected together and regarded as a whole, rather than individually and discretely as they have in most previous scholarship, these events demonstrate a pattern of thinking and behavior we have not heretofore attributed to Britons. While I do not wish to underestimate the extent to which conventional considerations of power informed the incidents I treat in the book, or to suggest that they had never before seen their like, I do maintain that unlike earlier instances of violence committed against national or colonial subjects, a substantial portion of Britons thought and acted in the extreme ways they did in the interwar period in an effort to repair the damage done to the individual and national psyche by deep and abiding personal suffering.

My arguments draw on the suggestions of a number of scholars who have attempted to connect the cultural with the political, the individual with the collective in their efforts to understand the psychological, emotional, and aesthetic appeal of fascism in Germany. The attraction of Nazism was not so much to be found in the political ideology it put forward as in its promise to obliterate the "emotions, images, and phantasms" that haunted the survivors of the war, to make whole the psyche fragmented by the experiences of war. Versions of the terrors and fears "that had provided the sociopsychological foundations of German fascism," as one literary critic put it—the psychic material that prepared the ground for the emergence of fascism—existed in virtually all those European societies that fought in the Great War. Britons played out the same emotional dynamics as Germans in the interwar period, but they did so in different ways, seeking the psychological solace that fascism offered without necessarily embracing the political doctrine. The assertion that it was at a "deep level of identity formation that Nazism was able to exert its most powerful appeal in its mobilization of the population, that the particular modes of address it deployed found their deepest resonances" applies to Britons, too, if we substitute for "Nazism" the campaigns directed against those depicted as "unEnglish."[14]

One way of staving off the terrors of shattering, fragmentation, and dissolution lay in lashing out against those forces that appeared to threaten the individual, to establish barriers against and distance between oneself and the threatening object. Trauma consists of the "obliteration of distinctions" that enable "things" and people to establish themselves as separate entities;[15] certainly, the language used by Britons of all creeds and convictions suggests a shared terror of boundary crossing, of the blurring of categories that establish identity and autonomy, and of the annihilation that must follow. Traumatized subjects, shattered subjects, must armor themselves against this threat of dissolution and annihilation; they often do so by perpetrating violence against those forces deemed to be threatening. The authoritarian figures thrown up by fascist regimes represent to these shattered subjects the force by means of which chaos and dissolution can be staved off; they provide coherent, unambiguous meanings and strong, absolute boundaries between self and threatening "other."[16]

Shell-shocked Britons sought to recreate a sense of wholeness, to resist the sensations of disruption, to fill in the gaps and erase the visions that threatened to tear them apart, to annihilate them. The process of making whole appears most often to take place through the telling of a story, a narrative or history that connects past with present, that mends the ruptures and fills in the gaps produced by the traumatic event. Progress toward recovery from trauma requires the individual victim to construct a coherent story comprised of prewar whole self, traumatized fragmented self, and recovered, integrated self. The stories of individuals traumatized by the war began to appear in Britain in 1928 with the arrival of the war memoir and war novel. Works by Richard Aldington, Siegfried Sassoon, Robert Graves, Edmund Blunden, Vera Brittain, Radclyffe Hall, and countless others followed the narrative structure of putting the disconnected pieces together to create a single, seemingly seamless, certainly comprehensible story of prewar, wartime, and postwar self and society, stories that, as one historian has shown, differed in significant ways from accounts of the same events recorded in their diaries at the time they occurred.[17]

British society, too, turned to a story of the war to effect its collective recovery; banishing the agonies of psychic shattering from collective consciousness involved adopting certain narratives about Englishness that served to make the psyche whole and establish clear and firm boundaries between self and other. The story of the Great War differed according to the interests of those mobilizing it to claim ownership of or membership in the nation. Common features populated the variety of versions: the war was fought to defend the nation and the empire, to uphold democracy and the rule of law, and to protect small nations from "Prussianism;" it was fought splendidly both at home and at the front by men and women of all stations who submerged their differences in a unified effort on behalf of the nation as a whole, who never gave a thought to giving in, who sacrificed their lives, their loved ones, their material comfort for the British nation and British empire; and for all that, all men and (some) women had earned the right to vote for the nation they had defended so well, and all Britons deserved a society befitting the sacrifices they had made on its behalf. The nation, and the political authority that serves and manipulates it, derives its justification for existence and its resilience from "the way in which it invokes its memories, and with what it remembers and why." Traumatic memories play a central role in the establishment and/or maintenance of political authority: in the case of rituals of remembrance or commemoration, for instance, the narrative of heroic sacrifice on behalf of the nation operates to sustain a powerful state. But traumatic memories can also destabilize, disrupt linear narratives that serve a particular social ordering; they open up possibilities for alternative orderings that might threaten political authority.[18] Narratives about the sacrifices made on behalf of the nation by women and by the working classes, for example, might be utilized to demand universal manhood and/or women's suffrage or to embarrass a government that is unable or unwilling to honor its promise of "a home fit for heroes." Struggles for control over these narratives involve numerous participants and interest groups; they are struggles for power in which questions of national belonging loom large. Within the basic outline of the narrative of the war, all sorts of questions were glossed over or never asked: who is the nation, after all, and what is its relationship to the empire? Whose democracy is to be upheld and whose pretentions to democracy assailed? Which small nations deserve protection from Prussianism and which do not? What of those people who did not behave splendidly, who broke down in terror or cowardice, who prospered at the expense of those who fought or lost? Were the sacrifices made at home and those at the front commensurate, and what were the costs of those sacrifices for individuals from a variety of stations, for their families, and for their country? Who would pay those costs? And who would decide these issues, in light of a newly enlarged and unpredictable electorate?

The peaceable flight to domesticity, to "quietude" and "safety first," as Conservatives were calling for as early as 1922,[19] offered one way to address the question of national belonging. The abandonment of a broad "British" identity for a smaller "English" identity on the part of many citizens, observed by Peter Mandler and others, involved pulling back from European, world, and imperial affairs and focusing on a much narrower field of view; it necessarily entailed the creation of a new national character. Mandler attributes the forging of a new "Englishness" to "a much greater sense of unity and stability among the survivors" and the wise leadership of Baldwin, who "set about painting a picture of the English national character that might be reassuring to Tories, familiar to Liberals, and perhaps even placatory to socialists." But the very construction of that national character, however "gentle and domesticated, kindly and humorous,"[20] required a mirror image, a foil, an "other" against which "Englishness" could be defined.

In the years immediately following the armistice in November 1918, Britons from all political quarters and ideologies began to categorize who did and did not belong to the nation, drawing lines according to race and ethnicity, class, and gender. The notion of "the nation" operated to naturalize a particular political and social ordering: the narrative of "the nation" as it served in and emerged from the Great War was used to close down a number of alternatives to or contestations of the social and political regime that went to war in 1914. Ultimately, Britons turned to narrating a particular story of themselves and their nation that responded to their needs to put the pieces back together, to reestablish wholeness, completeness, and continuity. This narrative, manifested in a number of political actions throughout the 1920s, cast a variety of groups as aliens who must be eliminated if the story of Englishness was to prevail and the individual and collective psyche repaired. Britons found relief from the terrors of dissolution and annihilation by fashioning a collective identity established against Irish Catholics, Jews, bolsheviks, Indians, West Indians, Africans, and, to a lesser extent, women and the working classes at home. Proceeding against these others—linguistically by categorizing them as enemies of the nation, but also materially through the visitation of great violence upon them in many instances—provided relief from the intolerable psychic conditions produced by horrific trauma and the inability to mourn unimaginable losses, and promised, however hollowly, to make the shattered subject whole. The existence of an empire containing a multitude of racial and ethnic peoples afforded the British an opportunity to work out their anxieties through violent actions that would not, ordinarily, be tolerated at home. In other words, the policies directed at and actions taken against aliens that were justified by the "extremes of Englishness"[21] did the psychic work that fascist ideology undertook abroad. Britain did not need a fascist government; its own politicians and government performed perfectly well in effecting the psychological, emotional, and cultural repair demanded by the devastations of the Great War.

1
Britons' Shattered Psyche

> The effect is to make the 'twenties seem not so much a period
> of history as an abnormal psychological state.[1]

The shell-shocked soldier—gendered male—has come to exemplify the
individual conditioned by the history of the twentieth century. The
Great War stands as the inaugural event of that century, establishing
the emotional states of the quintessential twentieth-century self that
subsequent wars, revolutions, and holocausts would intensify. The victim of a trauma whose scale and scope were unprecedented, whose
mind had been shattered by the endless cycles of bombardment, terror, destruction, and death, and whose control over mental and bodily
functions was shaky at best, the shell-shocked soldier came to represent
the subject of the age. For the "lost generation" and those who followed, shell shock provided the experience by means of which interwar
Britons—and here I want to emphasize women as well as men—came to
understand their sense of self, a reflection of the phenomenon anthropologist Jean Comaroff calls "cultural ontology." She asserts that people
in particular times and places arrive at various conceptualizations of
selfhood that make sense within the circumstances of those times and
places, that resonate with the social, economic, political, and cultural
practices that prevail. Karl Marx noted the same phenomenon when
he asserted that "production not only creates an object for the subject
but also a subject for the object," arguing that there is a relationship
between the external world and consciousness, or, as we might say
today, subjectivity.[2]
   Victorians embraced a version of subjectivity characterized in literature as the "divided self," a rational, moral, individualistic figure beset
by religious doubts, emotions, desires, and a sense of responsibility

to society that produced the sense of a two-sided personality. Beatrice Webb described this condition as "a continuous controversy between an Ego that affirms and an Ego that denies." Edwardians inherited some elements of the "divided self," but the literature of their period tended to stress inner unity, a state achieved by balancing various aspects of personality, of reconciling opposing selves and making them into an undivided whole. As E.M. Forster famously declared, "only connect," giving voice to the prevailing model of the mind as divided by competing tendencies but capable of unifying through the liberation of the subconscious. An "Edwardian synthesis" could readily be effected by bringing together two or even more elements of a single entity, by connecting them. Havelock Ellis' "painful sense of strain and division," "the dull aching tension" he felt between the pulls of science and spirituality were resolved when he adopted what he referred to as a religion of "life." "The two opposing psychic tendencies were fused in delicate harmony," he recalled. "My self was one with the Not-self, my will one with the universal will."[3]

The horrors of the Great War exploded this understanding of the mind as undivided self. The sights and experiences of war could not be integrated into customary patterns or meaning systems that organized the ordinary rhythms of life; they traumatized people. Because traumatic incidents are so overwhelming, so unprecedented, so horrifying in nature, they cannot fit within the narrative structure by means of which we make sense of ourselves and our lives. Instead, they are experienced as disruptions in the narrative stream, as gaps in the stories we use to define ourselves. Most often, victims and observers of or participants in unspeakable incidents attempt to suppress them, to bar their entry into consciousness, but such is the horrific nature of traumatic events that they cannot be fully denied. Memories of them insist on intruding into consciousness, but they do so not as a continuous, intelligible narrative that can be incorporated into one's recognizable life story, but in fragmented images or sensations that will not fit together to form a whole picture. Without a verbal, linear context into which the trauma can be assimilated and integrated, it will recur over and over again. The inability to construct a coherent narrative of the self in relation to the most extreme traumatic events, notes one scholar, may constitute "the true meaning of annihilation, for when one's history is abolished, one's identity ceases to exist as well." Shell shock promulgated a new sense of "self" and "self-awareness," compelling the emergence of a new subject, a new subjectivity, a subjectivity best characterized as shattered. Sufferers of shell shock frequently spoke of the fragmentation of their mental processes. An earlier sensation of psychic wholeness, autonomous separateness, continuity, meaning, and attachment had come apart, leaving a felt condition of rupture, disintegration, and shattering that threatened to leave the individual in pieces.[4]

The physical and psychic terrain of the twentieth century was dramatically transformed by the material and emotional traumas suffered during World War I and its immediate aftermath. The concept of Post-Traumatic Stress Disorder (PTSD) should not be understood to apply universally to regimes of trauma across time or space; PTSD is, rather, a particularly late-twentieth-century diagnosis arising out of political, social, and economic conditions of the time. We should insist on treating trauma historically, understanding its manifestations to be a product of the period and conditions of life from which it emerges. The association of trauma with mental injury emerged in the middle of the nineteenth century with the onset of railway accidents; it was extended to understand the mental states of soldiers who fought in the American civil war. These latter, however, produced representations that derived from the incidence of disease and untreated wounds, differing from those that would come later out of the trenches of the western front in World War I; the battles against the Germans and Japanese in World War II; the horrors of the Holocaust; and the jungles of Vietnam. In the case of the Great War, it was the blasted, splintered landscape of the trenches produced by constant shelling and the sight of bodies in pieces that provided the imagery through which the state of the mind in the postwar years would be represented and articulated.

The term shell shock derived from soldiers' exposure to massive artillery barrages. Producing extreme levels of ceaseless noise, they bombarded the senses with ear-splitting sound, light that turned night into day, and concussive force that knocked men down. As Ford put it in a letter to his daughter Katherine in December 1916, he was "blown up by a 4.2 & shaken into a nervous breakdown." Shells splintered trees and rent the landscape with their destructive force. The physical effects on the surrounding terrain produced by shellfire were consistently depicted in terms that evoked shattering. A Red Cross medic spoke of "fantastically splintered tree stumps," of shells fading away in "filmy shreds and tatters." German shells "ripped through the dark copse all about us, bursting in great rose-shaped splashes, green whirling vortices, up-sproutings, scatters and showers of unbearably brilliant flame." "Fragments of earth and stone tinkled on my helmet," he told his family. Lieutenant Bernard Pitt described in a letter of 31 March 1916, "a sight more shocking than the ruin of human work, a ghastly wood where broken trunks and splintered branches take on weird and diabolical forms." In a letter to his brother written in late July 1916, Lieutenant Christian Carver revealed that "one gets certain pictures absolutely engraved on one's soul . . . [During shelling], the familiar landscape showed up in fragments now here, now there, lighted by the blinding flash of the guns."[5]

What artillery did to earth and trees it also did to bodies. "Horses, men, women, and children blown to pieces," despaired Lance Corporal Harold Chapin to his wife in May 1915, as he recounted his work as a member of the Royal Army Medical Corps. Captain Theodore Wilson spoke in the spring of 1916 of "those poor torn bodies," of "the deliberate tearing of fine young bodies," of "that little singing splinter of metal" that wreaked such havoc, of "fine fellows ripped horribly out of existence by 'reeking shard.' " Private Thomas Dry wrote to his family from Egypt in January 1916, telling them of his experience digging out his comrades after an attack, describing "pieces of flesh, scalp, legs, tunics tattered and parts of soldiers carried away in blankets." Captain William Mason told of "the wounded whose flesh and bodies are torn in a way you cannot conceive," a sight shared by Ford Madox Ford as he watched "men, burst into mere showers of blood, and dissolving into muddy ooze." Sergeant-Major Frederic Keeling, in a letter to E.S.P. Haynes in March 1916, described his efforts to bring in a man wounded by shellfire. In a telling, if unconscious, association to the state of the soldier's body, he went on to ask Haynes if he had seen the exhibition of a set of drawings of shelling entitled *Fragments from France*.[6]

These images of fragments, splinters, and shards, of tearing and ripping, carried over to frontsoldiers' descriptions of their minds and mental states after too many days of shelling, wounds, and death. As Frederic Manning put it in his novel of the war, *Her Privates We*, when soldiers went into battle "the world would be shattered for them, and what was left of it they would have to piece together again, into some crazy makeshift that might last their time." Richard Aldington's protagonist George Winterbourne in *Death of a Hero* described trench life as a set of "circumstances which rent his mind to pieces." He described a particular battle as "a timeless confusion, a chaos of noise, fatigue, anxiety, and horror." He

> did not know how many days and nights it lasted, lost completely the sequence of events, found great gaps in his conscious memory. He did know that he was profoundly affected by it, that it made a cut in his life and personality. . . . His mind no longer wandered off

in long coherent reveries, but was either vaguely empty or thronged with too vivid memories.

Guy Chapman similarly spoke of the days just before the armistice in terms that evoked the disruption of thought, the gaps in memory that forbade a coherent telling of the experience. "The next six weeks remain in my memory a mere set of disconnected pictures with periods of complete blankness.... The cinematograph flicks past quickly. We had little understanding of the pictures."[7]

In four years of warfare, this small island nation of some 42 million people lost 750,000 men. Six million English, Welsh, Scottish, and Irish men served in the armed forces between 1914 and 1918; one in eight of them lost their lives. A total of 1.6 million servicemen—one in every four—suffered wounds or illnesses. Some 15,000 ships' passengers and crew members of merchant and fishing vessels died, and 1266 civilians were killed during air raids or bombardments from the sea.[8] Adding to the unspeakable combat deaths, an additional 250,000 people perished within six months in the influenza epidemic that swept through Great Britain in 1918 and 1919. Three millions Britons suffered the loss of a parent, spouse, sibling, or child, and many endured multiple deaths; even if they avoided the loss of a family member, few escaped first-hand knowledge of dead or maimed friends, neighbors, or co-workers.[9] As journalist Philip Gibbs observed,

> England was all in—all her men, all her women, and no escape for any of them in the service of death. No living body in England was exempt from the menace of destruction. Death came out of the skies, and chose old men and women, nursing mothers, babies, anyone. The enemy attacked them in little homes in back streets, in big factory centres, in the heart of London.

"It was a terrible war," asserted Ivy Compton-Burnett. "It got into every life, it got into every home."[10] On both the individual and the societal level, Britons were faced with the overwhelming task of mourning their dead, work that was often obstructed by spoken and unspoken injunctions against expressions of grief and by the very public memorials and national rituals that were intended to assuage it, forcing the feelings of sadness, pain, rage, abandonment, and disorientation that grief entails to find outlets elsewhere.

So much death could not have failed to wreak havoc on the psyches of millions of Britons, inducing in them something of the same kinds of emotional trauma incurred by men on the battlefield. "The war annihilated everyone and everything outside it," recalled Caroline Playne;[11] one need not make invidious comparisons between the experiences of civilian men, women, and children and the extreme conditions faced by combat soldiers to appreciate the agonies that confronted virtually all Britons, civilian and uniformed alike. Some 500,000 soldiers suffered extreme wounds in the war; 240,000 of them lost limbs; 10,000 lost their sight; and serious respiratory illnesses caused by gas warfare and generally deplorable conditions in the trenches afflicted about 55,000 veterans.[12] The official reports of 80,000 "shell-shocked" soldiers vastly underestimate the incidence of serious emotional trauma among the armed forces. Even if we limit—wrongly—our attributions of shell shock to the two-thirds of the six million men in uniform who served in the infantry,[13] where they witnessed or partook of incidents of the utmost horror, and allow that their exposure to such sights induced in them some measure of emotional trauma, then we are confronted by a significant population of individuals suffering from the phenomenon. If we add to them the friends and families of those who were killed or wounded, sometimes in the most hideous fashion, or who died of influenza, we arrive at a number of seriously traumatized individuals who, collectively, begin to constitute a "society," a "polity," a "nation."

Much of what we understand about the nature of post-traumatic stress disorder derives from the testimony of World War I veterans, front soldiers who witnessed and experienced the singular terrors of that war. But it was not just combat soldiers who reeled under the impact of the great conflict. Just as the condition of shell shock revealed that men could become hysterical—that is, like women—the events of the war demonstrated that women, like soldiers, could be shell-shocked. Noncombatants shared the devastation and sense of loss experienced by men on the battlefield, though perhaps not with the same intensity or degree of horror. Air raids and the shelling of cities, while infrequent by the standards of World War II, terrorized those who felt or saw their effects. Nurses, members of the Voluntary Aid Detachments (VADs), ambulance drivers, munitions workers, readers of letters home, and recipients of the dreaded news of a loved one's death at the front—all these civilians, men and women alike, faced the kinds of events, sights, and emotional assaults that might traumatize even the most steady of individuals.

The German bombardment of West Hartlepool, Whitby, and Scarborough from the sea in mid-December 1914, resulting in 700 casualties, shocked the inhabitants of those towns. Sylvia Pankhurst reported the distress this shelling caused to one woman: "it had terrified her inexpressibly and had seemed to last for years. People could not sleep now; many would not even go to bed. Everyone had a bundle made up in readiness for flight." In May 1915, Zeppelin raids on the East End of London killed seven civilians and injured 35 more. Nine other Zeppelin raids on the country occurred between June and October of 1915, killing 127 and wounding 352 Britons. Mrs A. Burnett Smith watched a Zeppelin raid in which her house was bombed. "To me it was a stupendous moment," she wrote in 1918,

> during which the whole fabric of existence seemed to be tottering— and we on the edge of some unimaginable abyss…. It was all so quick and so terrible, that we felt it must be the end of the world, the total destruction of everything we had considered stable in our earthly life.

When the bombing stopped, the noise of the explosions was "replaced by the cries of excited people, and the moans of the hurt and dying in the street." The experience stunned her, preventing her from sleeping and rattling her to the core. "I was the slave of physical fear after the excitement had died down," she recalled, "shaking in every limb, even to my lips." Her fear turned to grief that "tears you in a thousands ways." Finally she recognized that "my job is to gather up the fragments."[14]

Raids over London by German aircraft in the autumn of 1917 caused great destruction and produced deep-seated fear among the civilian population. In East London, 16 children were killed and 30 badly wounded by a bomb that landed on the school in whose cellar they had sought shelter. At Liverpool Station that same day, 146 people died and some 400 were injured in the raid,[15] an event that "under normal circumstances," Siegfried Sassoon, who witnessed it, observed, "would be described as an appalling catastrophe." He witnessed "horrified travelers… hurrying away" from the death and destruction wrought by the bombs that fell on the station. "While I stood wondering what to do," he recalled, "a luggage trolley was trundled past me; on it lay an elderly man, shabbily dressed, and apparently dead." Accustomed to the carnage of the trenches, Sassoon could not easily assimilate the danger faced by these ordinary civilians going about their daily routines. "This sort of danger," he allowed, "seemed to demand a quality of courage dissimilar to front line fortitude," where

> one was acclimatized to the notion of being exterminated and there was a sense of organized retaliation. But here one was helpless; an

invisible enemy sent destruction spinning down from a fine weather sky; poor old men bought a railway ticket and were trundled away again dead on a barrow; wounded women lay about in the station groaning.

The air raids provoked great anxiety, leading East End families, who suffered a disproportionate amount of the bombing, to sleep in the underground tube tunnels in anticipation of the attacks. Caroline Playne, somewhat insulated by virtue of her class status from the dangers experienced by inhabitants of the East End, nevertheless shared in "the dread and depression then everywhere prevailing." The complacency felt by Britons owing to their isolation from the continent received a staggering blow by these incursions. As Gibbs put it,

> England was no longer safe in her island. An island people, uninvaded for a thousand years, with utter reliance on her fleet as an invincible shield, were suddenly shocked into the knowledge that the sea about them was no longer an impassable gulf between them and all foreign foes. It was a shock which broke up the old psychology. We have not recovered from it yet, nor ever shall do.[16]

Women attending wounded soldiers confronted fearsome sights, sounds, and smells. Joan, the protagonist of Irene Rathbone's autobiographical novel, witnessed ghastly cases in her capacity as a VAD in France: "limbs which shrapnel had torn about and swollen into abnormal shapes, from which yellow pus poured when the bandgages were removed, which were caked with brown blood, and in whose gangrenous flesh loose bits of bone had to be sought for painfully with probes." During the battle for Passchendaele, recalled a member of the Women's Auxiliary Army Corps (WAAC) assigned to a dressing station, "troops came pouring up... and as rapidly as they went up they would be brought back—what was left of them—mangled masses of blood, bits of men, limbs missing, groaning bodies with intestines visible, sometimes khaki shapes that screamed like maniacs when the stretchers were lifted out."[17] Nurses, VADs, orderlies, and ambulance drivers repeatedly testified to the numbness with which they carried out their gruesome tasks by day, and the horrors that haunted their dreams by night.

Women in munitions factories faced the dangers common to heavy industrial work usually undertaken by men. Machines might cut off the fingers or rip off the scalps of women who did not give their whole concentration to their work; overhead crane drivers sometimes met their maker in fatal accidents. Factory explosions, which largely went unreported in the press owing to the prohibitions of the Defense of the Realm Act (DORA), occurred with greater frequency than the general public ever knew, and took the lives of hundreds of workers. Injuries sustained in these explosions could be counted in the thousands. One woman recalled an incident that took place in her factory in April of 1917: "some flames started coming along the line towards us, and two men in the shop got hold of us and threw us outside onto the grass.... The alarm was going and Queenie, our supervisor, had to go back for her watch. She was blown to pieces." Lottie Barker, a worker in the No. 6 National Shell Filling Factory near Nottingham, recounted hearing and feeling the 1 July 1918 blast that killed 134 people. "What a scene of horror met us," she recalled. "Men, women and young people burnt, practically all their clothing burnt, torn and dishevelled, their faces black and charred, some bleeding with limbs torn off, eyes and hair literally gone."[18]

The millions of people who could only guess at the fate of their neighbors, friends, and loved ones serving at the front suffered acute stress as they scanned the endless casualty lists or awaited the dreaded ringing of the door bell that would announce the death of their son, brother, husband, or father. Inexpressible grief confronted civilians as they received word of the deaths of their friends and family members. Months and years of anxiety could not prepare parents for the loss of their sons. Upon reading the telegram announcing the death of her son, Harold, Storm Jameson's mother "made the inhuman sound women make when they lose a son, a cry torn from the empty womb." Jameson could not comfort her mother, for whom her son's loss "had been an end for her, a hard and bitter end of her deep life." When Ivy Compton-Burnett's brother, Noel, died at the Somme, his widow tried to kill herself and had to be committed to a nursing home. Two of his sisters' suicide attempts succeeded. For Ivy, the personal tragedy of the war "quite smashed my life up, it quite smashed my life up." "I am a living witness of this crushing lifless [sic] stagnation of the spirit," she wrote shortly after the armistice. Burnett Smith's thoughts upon hearing that her friend had been killed on the Somme stood in for millions of others who suffered the same wounds of the heart "for which there could never be any cure this side of the grave." She, like Compton-Burnett, Vera Brittain, and millions of others, "nearer the breaking point than I knew," took the news like a body blow that laid her out flat. "When I got to bed there I found I was not able to get up again." Hilda Doolittle, who delivered her stillborn child in May of 1915, attributed the child's death to the war. "I had lost the ... [baby] in 1915 from shock and repercussions of war news broken to me in a rather brutal fashion," she recounted. Katherine Mansfield "was haunted by the news of her brother's death, and found she could not stop herself imagining the sights of war. 'I keep seeing all these horrors,' she wrote in 1918, 'bathing in them again and again (God knows I don't want to).' " For some, refusal to confront the pain of their losses offered the only way of surviving. Vera Brittain found that her "only hope" after the deaths of her fiancé, her friends, and her brother "was to become the complete automaton. . . . Thought was too dangerous," she said. "If once I began to think out exactly why my friends had died ... quite dreadful things might suddenly happen."[19]

The affective reticence characteristic of Britons, joined with public calls for the bereaved not to wear mourning clothes—"in England," Playne explained, "outward signs of mourning were taboo"—compelled many to bury their grief and put a good face on things, compounding the damage done by the deaths of their loved ones. Officially discouraged from expressing their grief for fear of contributing to the demoralization of the country in wartime, parents who had lost their children, in particular, found themselves under the most terrible stress imaginable. What historian Adrian Gregory describes as the "denial of death" issued in a new emotional regime, "a changed set of parameters in the psychological possible." "Women crushed down their repulsions, their sorrows and anxieties," declared Playne,

> and deadened their souls by ceaseless activities. Still, with all the determination in the world, war brought sorrows that could not be denied or brushed away. So that when the gnawing of some sudden unbearable grief, some irrefutable blow, struck down women at home, the tortured mind found refuge, now and again, in real dementia. Fantastic imaginings were adopted and substituted for obvious truths.[20]

Numerous civilians sought treatment for the symptoms of war neuroses and were recognized as suffering from such by medical authorities. *The Lancet* registered in October 1915 the admission of a woman to Leicester Mental Hospital as a direct result of war news: five of her seven sons at the front had been wounded. The Dorset County Asylum reported that "stress was frequently a well-recognised cause of mental breakdown, and that not a few cases were associated with the war, both among the wives of soldiers and young recruits." By March 1916, *The Lancet* had come to accept the reality of civilian war neuroses, arguing that "while the stress of war on the soldier is discussed, it should not be forgotten that the nervous strain to which the civilian is exposed may require consideration and appropriate treatment." Symptoms of war shock among civilians were "by no means uncommon," it conceded. Mary Dexter, training at the Medica-Psychological Clinic, treated a number of women for war neuroses in 1917, among them a nurse and a munitions worker—"an hysterical girl." Other girls, one "mad with nerves" and another suffering from "conversion hysteria," sought her help at the clinic. One writer, in *The Problem of Nervous Breakdown* (1919), tried to counter the growing conviction that the war had produced a nation of neurotics, but even he conceded that civilians caught up in the violence presented some of the symptoms of "shell-shock of the battlefield."[21]

The emotional fallout of the war was compounded by the flu epidemic that swept into Britain in the last months of it, dealing the war-weary populace a cruel blow. It wreaked its havoc on military and civilian populations in three waves, the first in June and July of 1918, the second in October and November of 1918, and the third in February 1919. The incidence, symptomology, and mortality rates of the flu exacerbated the traumas of wartime, extending to the home front an immediate and direct experience of widespread misery and death.

The flu killed over 30 million people throughout the world. George Newman, Chief Medical Officer of Great Britain's Ministry of Health, called it "one of the great historic scourges of our time, a pestilence which affected the well-being of millions of men and women and destroyed more human lives in a few months than did the European war in five years." It appeared with explosive suddenness, and "simply had its way. It came like a thief in the night and stole treasure." Doctors estimated that 800 of 1000 persons contracted only a mild case of the flu; but of the other 200 severely afflicted, some 80 percent of them died.[22] Great Britain suffered perhaps 250,000 losses, one-third of the numbers killed during the war. The newspaper columns listing the number of dead from flu began to rival and even outpace those listing the numbers of dead from the war.

The nature of this particular strain of influenza defied all previous understandings of the disease. It struck quickly and without warning, felling people in their homes, in schools, in stores and businesses, and in the streets. Unlike its predecessors, which tended to take infants and the elderly, this strain preferred men and women aged 15–45, victims in the prime of their lives, like those struck down in the trenches. Medical authorities could not explain this "peculiar character" of age distribution of mortality, a phenomena that contributed to the sense of utter incomprehension the disease produced throughout all segments of society. This was an illness without precedent, whose etiology and treatment could not be discerned or determined.

The nature and scope of the flu compelled medical authorities to abandon their ordinarily clinical accounts and describe the situation in highly charged, graphic language. Herbert French recounted what he believed to be a typical situation. "In the midst of perfect health in a circumscribed community," he wrote,

> such as a barracks, or a school, the first case of influenza would occur, and then within the next few hours or days a large proportion—and occasionally even every single individual of that community—would be stricken down with the same type of febrile illness, the rate of spread from one to another being remarkable. The patient would be seized rapidly, or almost suddenly, with a sense of such prostration as to be utterly unable to carry on with what he might be doing; from sheer lassitude he would be obliged to lie down where he was, or crawl with difficulty back to bed.

The Lancet abandoned its scientific distance when it described the flu's "invasion of every hitherto safe nook and cranny in the inhabited world."[23] Barracks became converted to sick rooms overnight, hospitals became so overrun with patients that they had to turn new arrivals away. Nurses and doctors could not handle the unprecedented numbers of cases; undertakers could not fill the orders for caskets that came streaming in nor gravediggers handle the volume requesting their services.

The epidemic took on the countenance of Britain's battlefield enemy. For some, the war was incorporated in their hallucinations stemming from the disease. The *Daily Express* cited an inquest report on a nine-year-old boy whose death from the flu followed a delirious episode when he "jumped out of bed, swinging his arms about and saying he was fighting the Germans." For others, the war served as an obvious metaphor. In October 1918, a physician told an inquest panel that doctors were "fighting at home a foe as bad as the Huns." Stories about the "Influenzal Hun" who attacked innocent victims appeared in newspaper accounts. An advertisement in the *Illustrated London News* warned that the flu placed Britons "under the domination of enemies more ruthless and destructive even than the Hun." The copy spoke of " 'Germ-Huns' in their trenches" against whom the product touted—Kruschen Salts—"is your first line of defence." A reporter for the *Daily Express* told of his visit to a London hospital "to inspect a party of the enemy who had been taken captive...and were at the time interned in the 'cage' of a microscope. They wore a pink uniform," he noted. Gas masks were urged on the populace; indeed, doctors and scientists allowed as how "the lesions produced by poisonous gases during the last war resembled those seen in the respiratory complications of influenza." Doctors, asserted the *British Medical Journal* in April 1919, who "set out to conquer [the influenza] disease have mightier opponents than Ludendorff or Hindenburg, and must face a longer campaign than that of 1914–1918."[24]

This strain of influenza produced in many of its victims a variety of vivid and frightening physical symptoms that had not been encountered in previous incarnations of the disease. Doctors reported some patients who "spit up a quantity of frothy sputum tinged with bright blood." "The dreaded blueness" of the face caused by heliotrope cyanosis disturbed observers, lay persons and physicians alike, who cited the incidence of this particular manifestation repeatedly. "The purple-black skin was terrifying to everyone," wrote Eileen Pettigrew. The British Ministry of Health's official report on the flu included in its pages color illustrations of the shockingly purple faces of patients suffering from "this dreaded heliotrope cyanosis." It was this symptom that signalled almost certain death, doctors came to understand. "It was amongst cases of this type that the great mortality of the epidemic occurred," observed the Ministry of Health physicians. "In going round a large ward, one could, without examining the patients at all beyond looking at their countenances, pick out those who were going to die with almost uniform certainty by reason of their colour alone."[25]

The flu left survivors with a variety of mental symptoms, many of them represented by physicians and the press in terms similar to those used to describe sufferers of shell shock. As Caroline Playne put it, "the universal neurosis which endangered human society" during the war had "its analogy...in the plague of nervous character" following the onslaught of influenza. Pronounced fatigue, lassitude, depression, sleeplessness, hallucinations, emotional lability, and even dissociation accompanied the physical debilitation of the disease. Dr G. Holliday wrote to the *British Medical Journal* on 17 August 1918 that "mental symptoms were frequent" in the cases he saw; Samuel West informed readers of *The Lancet* on 1 February 1919 that "the depression which follows influenza is so constant that it ought to be regarded as part of the disease." The medical correspondent for *The Times*, having contracted the illness himself, advised readers that "the most distressing symptom was a swift loss of mental capacity and then inability to think coherently." "All forms of hysteria have been observed after influenza," reported Thomson and Thomson in 1919, "such as hysterical convulsions and the so-called hystero-epilectic attacks." "Post-influenzal neurasthenia is very familiar," they noted, "post-influenzal psychoses" "frequently observed and reported." They cited a study that asserted that influenza, "of all the infectious diseases . . . is the most likely to be followed by mental disorder." *The Lancet* declared in December 1918 that "the 'higher centres' [of the nervous system] suffer chiefly. Marked depression is common, emotional instability is often seen, and suicide is by no means rare."[26]

Ivy Compton-Burnett came down with the flu in the summer of 1918 and was discovered by mere chance lying unconscious on the floor of her flat. She exhibited delirium and, when recovered from the acute stage of the disease, "extreme debility, unable to read or write." She asked to be read to, but could not tolerate much stimulus, asking her sister to "read, but don't put any expression into it. Read in a dull, monotonous voice." She took up mindless tasks as her recovery progressed, but "I couldn't do brainwork," she explained.[27]

In Katherine Anne Porter's fictional account of the flu epidemic, her protagonist, Miranda, contracts the flu, becoming delirious and hallucinating scenes that explicitly recalled the war. She believed she saw her physician killing a child in a set of horrifying images.

> Across the field came Dr Hildesheim, his face a skull beneath his German helmet, carrying a naked infant writhing on the point of his bayonet, and a huge stone pot marked Poison in Gothic letters. He stopped before the well that Miranda remembered in a pasture on her father's farm, . . . and into its pure depths he threw the child and the poison, and the violated water sank back soundlessly into the earth. Miranda, screaming, ran with her arms over her head; her voice echoed and came back to her like a wolf's howl, Hildesheim is a Boche, a spy, a Hun, kill him, kill him before he kills you.

In an episode of dissocation, Miranda described how "her mind, split in two, acknowledged and denied what she saw in the one instant, for across an abyss of complaining darkness her reasoning coherent self watched the strange frenzy of the other coldly, reluctant to admit the truth of its visions, its tenacious remorses and despairs."[28]

At the age of two, Anthony Burgess was found by his father lying on his cot in the same room where his mother and sister had lain dead for an unknown period of time. In a passage recalling the gaps in memory opened up by traumatic events, Burgess remembered an early period of his life "sitting on a shoulder in Manchester's Piccadilly while a flag-waving crowd cheers the Armistice. Then the lights go out." The death of his mother and sister remained blank in his mind, but he sometime later "came to full consciousness in a terraced house...in the care of my mother's sister." In language significant for its imagery of the war, he added, "opposite the house was a great infirmary where, I learned, people were cut open. This gratuitous slashing and slitting seemed reasonable to me, who must have absorbed by osmosis the ethos of the times." The "cutting up of living bodies" haunted his dreams and perhaps his waking hallucinations as he lay in bed under a picture of a gypsy woman. "When I thought I was asleep the picture would open on loud hinges and disclose the world of cutting up live but uncomplaining bodies," he recounted. "It was lighted by fire. I was given the choice of joining the bodies or else remaining where I was, in the big lumpy flock bed which was steadily filling with horse shit...The turds were turning into aromatic serpents with teeth." That time, he wrote, was one of "fragments" with "little meaning. There is murk with occasional dull flashes of things and people. It is the lack of continuity that disconcerts, as though one were perpetually dying and being reborn to trivialities." He spoke of his mother having "joined the great boneyard of the war and its aftermath." He later attributed the emotional coldness of his fictional characters to his having lost the affection of his mother at so young an age.[29]

Shell shock afflicted not simply individuals or groups of individuals, but the whole of British society. Psychiatrist Judith Herman notes that

> there is a simple, direct relationship between the severity of the trauma and its psychological impact, whether that impact is measured in terms of the number of people affected or the intensity and duration of harm.... the greater the exposure to traumatic events, the greater the percentage of the population with symptoms of post-traumatic stress disorder.

It is not just that large numbers of individuals have been afflicted by devastating events; traumatized societies are not merely collections of traumatized people. Rather, notes one sociologist, "traumatic wounds inflicted on individuals can combine to create a mood, an ethos—a group culture, almost, that is different from (and more than) the sum of the private wounds that make it up. Trauma, that is, has a social dimension." Communities, like individuals, assaulted by multiple blows of pain, grief, and terror are those whose entire outlook has been altered: "they look out at the world through a different lens," they possess "a changed *worldview*." What theorist Cathy Caruth calls the "radical disruption and gaps of traumatic experience" mirror the sense Britons had that the war had produced a gulf between one world prior to the war and another after it. Moreover, the mechanisms by which traumatized individuals seek to escape the agonies of their memories may be utilized by larger collectivities as well. "Denial, repression, and dissociation operate on a social as well as an individual level," observes Herman.[30]

The images of the Great War—of the industrial onslaught of heavy artillery upon the physical landscape and, most importantly, on the minds and bodies of the men in the trenches—provided a template of sorts for organizing oneself in relation to the world that differed from earlier manifestations of trauma, such as those from railway accidents or the American civil war, for example. Neurobiologists have found that the brain re-constructs its "architecture" as new experiences registered through the eyes or the ears or other sensory organs are gathered and ordered in certain groups of interconnected cells; over time, the sensory input of images or experiences is categorized into "schemes" or patterns into which the mind seeks to place new information or sensory input. "With sufficient experience, the brain comes to contain a model of the world," states W.H. Calvin, a model that operates to organize memories according to its pre-existing structures. One's relationship to those memories, fitting into a pattern informed by the visual images of shattered, fragmented things and people, trauma theorists argue, constitutes one's identity, in effect. For memory, as Jeffrey Alexander reminds us, is "deeply connected to the contemporary sense of the self."[31]

Some neurobiologists suggest that images and the emotions they conjure can be transmitted from person to person, offering an explanation for how even individuals *not* connected with traumatic experiences might incorporate the images and emotions of those who were. Other theorists have identified as "a secondary traumatic stressor" the mere hearing about or learning of other people's traumas. Described as "emotional contagion" or "a form of empathy," this secondary trauma can have a profound impact on those who witness the suffering of others and produce in the witness many of the same symptoms exhibited by the original trauma victim.[32] The insights of these neurobiologists explain how the changes involved in societies moving from one model of "cultural ontology" to another may take place. After all, Hilda Doolittle's recounting of the loss of her baby suggests that it was "*not a* response to direct violence. It was a story which did the damage."[33] The images of wartime and the model of the mind as shattered, experienced by millions of people, may have been sufficiently contagious to produce a whole society—already reeling with unbearable grief and loss—with similar visions and understandings of the nature of the self, however unconscious they might have been.

Certainly this imagery of shattering informed popular renditions of the post war mind. As we have seen, combat veterans represented their minds as fragmented and shattered in the memoirs that poured forth beginning in 1928. Popular fiction incorporated this model in a number of characters as well, beginning as early as 1919. Rebecca West's returning soldier, the shell-shocked Chris Baldry, for instance, had abandoned in his mind his current life and returned to a time 15 years earlier, stranding his cousin and his wife Kitty in the present and taking up with his former love, Margaret. His cousin, the narrator, imagines his choice of Margaret over her and Kitty in terms of two crystal balls, in one of which Margaret resided, the other of which contained her and Kitty. "He sighs a deep sigh of delight and puts out his hand to the ball where Margaret shines," wrote West. "His sleeve catches the other one and sends it down to crash in a thousand pieces on the floor.... No one weeps for this shattering of our world." Dorothy Sayers, whose husband returned from the war shell shocked, gave Peter Wimsey and many of the suspects who peopled her crime stories the same history. All of her early mysteries contain one or more shell-shocked character; as one figure puts it,

> Here we've been and had a war, what has left 'undreds o' men in what you might call a state of ekilibrium. They've seen all their friends blown up or shot to pieces.... They may seem to forget it and go along as peaceable as anybody to all outward appearance, but it's all artificial, you get my meaning. Then, one day, something 'appens to upset them ... and something goes pop inside their brains and makes raving monsters of them. It's all in the books,

he adds, offering an explanation for the widespread adoption of the mind in pieces as archetypal interwar subject. Lord Peter himself had been "blown up and buried in a shell-hole" in 1918, returning home with "a bad nervous breakdown, lasting, on and off, for two years. After that, he set himself up in a flat in Piccadilly ... and started out to put himself together again." He turned to detective work for distraction, but the occupation served rather to exacerbate his mental condition. As his uncle observed, "Peter's intellect pulled him one way and his nerves another, till I began to be afraid they would pull him to pieces. At the end of every case we had the old nightmares and shell-shock again."[34]

Female protagonists in popular novels also suffered from war trauma and exhibited a similar mental condition of disconnection, dissociation, and fragmentation. "Scrap," the suggestively nicknamed character in Elizabeth von Arnim's *The Enchanted April* (1922), felt herself destroyed by the war. "The war finished Scrap," wrote Arnim. "It killed the one man she felt safe with." A persistent "noise" in her head crowded out any possibility of thinking coherently. Her mind "clogged," she sought quiet that might enable her to "really clear up her mind; really come to some conclusion.... almost any conclusion would do; the great thing was to get hold of something, catch something tight, cease to drift." Like a piece of paper blown about from place to place, Scrap could not settle or find mooring. Her "attention wouldn't stay fixed;" her "mind slipped sideways." Rose Macaulay's 1919 *What Not, A Prophetic Comedy* declared that wars "put a sudden end to many of the best intellects, the keenest, finest minds, which would have built up the shattered ruins of the world in due time. And many of the minds that are left are battered and stupefied." Her narrator saw around her people behaving "like a man long sick who has just begun to get about again and cannot yet make anything coherent of the strange, disquieting, terrifying... jumble which breaks upon his restored consciousness."[35]

In the years following the war and the onslaught of the influenza epidemic, the model of the mind conjured by Edwardians came apart. The enlightened male subject of prewar Western society—a rational, autonomous, and bounded whole—and his subsequent Freudian counterpart—a divided self driven by instincts and urges that were nevertheless contained within a stratified tripartite structure of id, ego, and superego—no longer proved adequate to the task of representing the subject of postwar Europe. Instead, the self theorized by Jacques Lacan served as a far more persuasive representative of the conditions and circumstances produced by the most terrible war to date, which was followed by an epidemic illness whose scope and behavior was unprecedented. Possessed of and by a shattered psyche and lacking control over both his bodily and mental capacities, the postwar masculine archetype, whose attributes should be extended to include women, was reflected in Lacan's conception of the true self as an irretrievable, inaccessible other. Where Freud posited that subjects attain a unified, if fraught, identity through the process of oedipal conflict, Lacan's theory of how the individual arrives at a sense of selfhood involved the infant perceiving himself [*sic*] in a mirror. The image of a whole self produced by the mirror, according to Lacan, conjures up the fantasy of a previous moment when the body was not whole, when it was in pieces, fragmented and fluid, vulnerable to drives that threatened to annihilate it. The ego, in this formulation, acts as a kind of armor designed to stave off the return of the body in pieces, to protect against the chaotic forces that might reduce the subject once again to fragmentation and dissolution. Those forces might be internal or external; they might be conscious or unconscious sexual desires, or racial, sexual, gendered, or political "others".[36]

This shattered subject armored against dissolution has a history; it is not, as Lacan would have it, a universal model constant across time and space. Rather, the twentieth-century subject reflects the traumas induced by the conditions and experiences of violence, death, and loss. It is an aggressive subject, whose very existence may depend on inflicting injury and even death upon those "others" who so threaten his psychic and bodily integrity. C. Fred Alford has argued in this regard that "hatred is egostructuring. It can define a self, connecting it to others, anchoring it in the world, while at the same time acting as a fortress."[37] We might, for example, understand the cruelty and violence of Anthony Burgess' *A Clockwork Orange* as a product of his efforts to defend himself, his ego, against the ravages of childhood trauma and grief that threatened to tear him apart.

Men and women returning from the theatre of war found themselves disoriented, confused, helpless, and useless. "You may say that everyone who had taken physical part in the war was then mad," wrote Ford Maddox Ford. "No one could have come through that shattering experience and still view life and mankind with any normal vision." Depression, lassitude, and indifference to danger, horrors, and death plagued many. "Life was pointless," wrote a soldier upon his return from the war. "Many of us were quite indifferent to the future," a sentiment echoed by C.E. Montague, who wrote of "the curious indifference in presence of public wrongs and horrors." Rathbone's autobiographical Joan, returning from work at the front, believed that if someone told her that "she would have to leave all this and die, she simply would have said, 'Oh!' At the roots of her being there lay a vast indifference."[38]

The year 1919 might have been "the maddest year of all," as one soldier put it, but veterans continued to experience traumatic symptoms well into the 1920s. Many could not throw off the sights and sounds of the war and suffered nightmares and flashbacks for months and even years. "Shells used to come bursting on my bed at midnight," recounted Robert Graves, even though his wife, "Nancy shared it with me; strangers in daytime would assume the faces of friends who had been killed." The sound of a car backfiring "would send me flat on my face, or running for cover," while lectures he attended at Oxford were often interrupted by scenes of battle. These flashbacks continued through 1928. Ford walked around feeling that "all things that lived and moved and had volition and life might at any moment be resolved into a scarlet viscosity seeping into the earth of torn fields."[39]

In part because they feared the nightmares that would follow sleep, insomnia haunted returning veterans. Some succumbed to amnesia—bouts of blackouts usually followed Graves' flashbacks. J.R. Ackerley felt enormous guilt that he had survived the war when his brother, Peter, had not. He found that he could not remember anything about the weeks he shared with his brother in the same battalion; his memory of other events and people was so bad, he allowed, that he could not say with any confidence that he really cared about anyone. A number of soldiers at the military hospital at Warrington "had returned from the war so utterly disturbed in mind and spirit that they had no sense at all of their own identity." Thousands more like them inhabited British "lunatic asylums." Others suffered delusions and hallucinations. Vera Brittain became obsessed by the belief that her face was changing, at one time sprouting a beard and at another turning into a witch. For 18 months, her delusions possessed her, bringing her to "the borderland of craziness."[40]

Returning soldiers, nurses, and ambulance drivers could not control their emotions; they felt hysterical, overwhelmed. As Rathbone described it,

> sometimes you felt quite ordinary... And suddenly, out of the four corners as it were, misery came, and swamped you. You could do nothing about it. You just sat at the heart of it. Everything else was blotted out—even your personality. You were just a primordial, enduring, suffering nerve. And then, after an hour, after a day—that sea withdrew; and you emerged, if not to life, to something that was tolerable.

Ackerley found himself pursuing sex obsessively, a compulsion he was not able to throw off until the 1940s. Some killed themselves: Bury men who had joined the Lancashire Fusiliers as a "pals brigade" suffered terrible losses to suicide. Shell-shocked men like James Scott, who cut his throat in the middle of the night, despite efforts by his mother and brother to keep their eye on him; or John Galloway, who jumped from the lavatory window of a hospital ward; or Bert Peachey, who hanged himself after a stint in the Prestwich Asylum, continued to take their lives right up to 1938.[41]

Returning from the war brought its own pain, especially for those who had found in the trenches a camaraderie they could find no where else. Bonded to one another through a literal ordeal of fire, these men shared emotions and experiences that no one who had not been through the war could understand, they believed. Leaving those comrades for peacetime existence produced a sense of disconnection from anything meaningful, and often produced a sense of alienation and atomization that plagued many veterans. Herbert Read recognized that "the sense of unity and of unanimity" fostered by the war could not survive demobilization, bemoaning the fact that "all that comradeship was to vanish once the storm was over" and soldiers returned to civilian life as "demobilized particles." Guy Chapman found that the men of his battalion "had become so much a part of me that its disintegration would tear away something I cared for more dearly than I could have believed. I was it, and it was I." Upon demobilization, he felt that "the whole of our world was crumbling," "our civilization was being torn in pieces before our eyes." The imagery of fragmentation and dissolution peppered their accounts of postwar life.[42]

Veterans, men and women alike, found that the society to which they returned could not or would not embrace them with the respect and dignity they believed their sacrifices had earned them. Some two-thirds of the unemployed in the early 1920s had been members of the armed forces.[43] Out of work, finding it difficult to adapt to civilian life, these one-time heroes were now "returned soldiers," "a problem to their country, if not a bore," as Rathbone noted. They "were a nuisance, and even a menace to everybody whose job was uncertain," declared Aldington, decrying the public's "indifference verging on hostility towards the men of the returning army." Where once "you were the savior of your country," now "you were a rotter who had acquired habits of idleness and insobriety in the King's service." Veterans especially resented the apparent failure of postwar society to appreciate the nature of those sacrifices, to ask them to go about their lives as if no traces of the wounds of war existed. The sense that civilians had forgotten and betrayed the sacrifices made by soldiers plagued many veterans, whose fury sometimes flared into uncontrollable rage. When Aldington learned of the desecration of skulls at Verdun, he "knew what it was to feel murder in one's heart," a situation, he believed, that "supplied the material from which fascists were made" on the continent. He feared no such danger in England, but in comparing the "unnecessary bitterness and misery" caused by the country turning its back on its returning vets to "the more acute form" of it on the continent, Aldington suggested that the difference was one of degree, not kind. Carrington put it more pointedly, declaring baldly that "all the elements that produced the phenomenon of fascism in Italy and Germany were at work in the other belligerent countries." This rage could—and in some instances, did—explode in violence, as was the case in the race riots in the summer of 1919 and in individual acts of assault committed by demobilized soldiers. Carrington described the "love for ganging-up with the other boys, a craving to demonstrate one's manliness, and a delight in anti-social violence" characteristic of returned soldiers, including himself. Gibbs believed that the "dreadful crimes, of violence and passion" on the part of soldiers or ex-soldiers that filled the newspapers derived from the hatred for the Germans instilled by four years of war, but we should probably understand the rage that "surge[d] up when there are no Germans present, but some old woman behind an open till, or some policeman ... or in a street riot where fellow-citizens are for the time being 'the enemy' " as manifestations of post-traumatic stress disorder.[44]

The anxieties, confusion, disorders, instability, dislocations, and divisions of the immediate postwar years engendered a number of responses at the level of both the individual and the collective. Individual veterans, male and female alike, produced narratives in a spate of poetry, war novels, and memoirs that appeared starting in 1928. Writing the narrative of their experiences enabled many veterans to put to rest the confusion and incoherence that haunted their lives. As Aldington put it, "By writing *Death of a Hero* I purged my bosom of perilous stuff which had been poisoning me for a decade. When I had finished, had said my say and cussed my cusses, I felt the lightness and tranquillity [*sic*] of a morning after a thunder storm." The upheaval and possibility of flooding represented by a thunder storm gave way to clarity and calm. It appears to have taken about ten years for returning vets to compose the narrative that adequately gave meaning to their experiences: Graves "made several attempts during [the twenties] ... to rid myself of the poison of war memories by finishing my novel, but had to abandon it." *Goodbye to All That* came out in 1929, part of that "flood of wartime reminiscences," as Carrington described it, that inundated the reading public. Ford's *No Enemy*, which appeared in 1929, was the means by which, as his biographer noted, he "was re-creating, in fact and literature, his own life, a process that could almost be described as natural psychotherapy." For some, a single memoir would not do; Siegfried Sassoon, for example, as Paul Fussell has observed, obsessively perseverated over the war, producing account after account that failed to put things to rest. Vera Brittain, arguably, did the same, with her series of "Testaments."[45]

Just as the war memoirs served the needs of individuals to place themselves within a coherent narrative stream, the overwhelming assaults on the nation—defying narration, as we have seen in the denial of grief and the obliteration of the flu epidemic from memory—created a desperate demand for a national narrative of wholeness. The yearning for unity permeated public discourse, especially that associated with the memorialization of Armistice Day and the Tomb of the Unknowns. Sir Percy Fitzpatrick, in suggesting that the country set aside 11 November as an official day of remembrance, observed that "when we are divided it may serve to remind us of the greater things we hold in common." The *Daily Express* used the occasion of that day in 1919 to urge that "there must be a truce in domestic quarrels, an end to industrial strife. We must all pull together lest the rewards of victory be thrown away." The *London Times Armistice Day Supplement* for 1920 described that year's service of remembrance in Westminster Abbey as a "proclamation, gladly made, that we are all equal, all members of one body, or rather one soul.... members of one orchestra,...one body politic." The War Graves Commission could not be budged from its determination that all of the Britons whose remains could be recovered from the battlefields of the war would be interred under monuments that were "uniform" in every detail. "What is done for one should be done for all," insisted the commission's chairman, as if the very unity of the nation, the survival of its "one immortal soul," depended upon it. Bob Bushaway has argued that the Armistice Day celebrations did effect the national integration they sought to create, dulling incipient political conflicts and paving the way for the emergence of moderate conservatism under Stanley Baldwin. Adrian Gregory offers a corrective to this view, arguing instead that the rituals of memorialization on Armistice Day, while they may have contributed to visions of unity in the nation, also created their own divisions. For commemoration can actually foreclose the very work of reconciliation with loss it seeks to effect. Drawing upon Freud's distinction between mourning and melancholia—mourning entailing successful grieving that enables an individual or group to move beyond its losses, on the one hand, while melancholia involves loss that is never put to rest but is a constant and ever-present intrusion in one's life— Larry Ray observes that some forms of commemoration stimulate not acceptance but anger, and may serve to justify vengeance against those perceived to be responsible for continuing hardship. "In a context of dramatic social upheaval," he believes, "communities can externalize dangerous experiences onto 'enemies' with whom they were previously intimate."[46]

In order for individuals and societies to begin their healing through the construction of narrative accounts that integrate traumatic experiences, a felt condition of safety must be established, and the two processes can take a long time; the ten year gap between the end of the war and the appearance of the war literature might be seen as the period in which that sense of safety and the coherent narrative developed. As Herman notes, recovery of a sense of self "depends upon a feeling of connection to others. The solidarity of a group provides the strongest protection against terror and despair, and the strongest antidote to traumatic experience. Trauma isolates; the group re-creates a sense of belonging." Thus, a second stage of recovery involves reconnection with the community from which one has become alienated or disconnected, and that process requires that the community "assign responsibility for the harm." British society as a whole constructed its coherent narrative through a variety of developments and events designed to tell a particular story of the nation, one that involved the separating out of forces to whom blame for British ills could be assigned so that safety could be established: Jews and blacks had behaved ignominiously during the war, seeking out refuge while native Britons conducted themselves with honor, and took jobs that rightfully belonged to returning soldiers; Irish and Indian nationals had betrayed the country by taking advantage of the war to advance their agendas for independence, and in the case of Ireland, the Easter Rising of 1916 had required a redeployment of troops badly needed at the front. Workers had undermined the recovery of the nation from the war with their selfish insistence on a living wage. Women had reveled in the freedoms and opportunities afforded them at the expense of frontsoldiers, and then refused to give up their jobs to returning soldiers; their demands for an equal franchise in place of the partial enfranchisement granted them in 1918 demonstrated a galling ingratitude. The felt condition of safety that would provide the space within which to construct a story of national identity and unity took some ten years to develop, during which time Britons identified and appeared to eliminate the threats from their presence.[47]

The structures of emotion generated by the tragedies of the Great War found expression in a variety of political incidents and events, to which individuals, government, and society as a whole responded in a variety of ways. In many of these incidents—the shootings at Amritsar, the race riots in the port towns, the actions of the Black and Tans and Auxiliaries in Ireland—individuals used or caused to be used physical violence against British colonial subjects. It is reasonable to see much of the violent behavior as the effects of trauma, as efforts on the part of the perpetrators to stave off, by lashing out against, potential boundary violations that threatened their psychic integrity. The actions of those individuals themselves generated a broader, societal response among the British public: in some instances, they excited a loud public outcry against them; in others, a confident approbation of the violence. It is in these responses that we can observe the attempts to forge a national identity—and therefore a national unity—by identifying those who must be expelled from society. That fashioning of national identity was a contested process—just what constituted Englishness was vigorously disputed, often along expected political lines, but sometimes not.

2
Jews, "Blacks," and the Promises of Radical Conservatism, 1919–1925

> Only by rigidly guarding his frontiers, and by restriction of immigration, can he preserve his race purity and save himself from extinction.[1]

The violence and upheaval of the Great War seemed to continue even after hostilities between Britain and Germany ceased in November 1918. Frontsoldiers returned home in a violent frame of mind. "All was not right with the spirit of the men who came back," Philip Gibbs wrote in 1920 of the veterans.

> Something was wrong. They put on civilian clothes again, looked to their mothers and wives very much like the young men who had gone to business in the peaceful days before August of '14. But they had not come back the same men. Something had altered in them. They were subject to queer moods, queer tempers, fits of profound depression alternating with a restless desire for pleasure. Many of them were easily moved to passion when they lost control of themselves. Many were bitter in their speech, violent in opinion, frightening.[2]

In January 1919, returning soldiers rioted all over England; in June 1919, soldiers waiting to be demobilized attacked the Epsom police station and killed the station sergeant; in July, ex-servicemen rioting in protest against having been excluded from the ceremonies that marked "Peace Day" in Luton destroyed the town hall, resulting in 100 casualties. Rathbone's fictional protagonist Joan, who went to work in a War Pensions Committee office after the war ended, observed that "to refuse a man his claim was a detestable task, and was often to provoke his

35

fury. . . . All the men seemed to be nervy, and some definitely unhinged. Doubtless they would settle down in time, but their release from the military machine was not, at the moment, beneficial to them." *The Vote*, a feminist paper, reported in May 1919 that "certain disquieting features marked the demonstration of the Discharged Soldiers and Sailors last Monday afternoon." It especially noted, with deep concern, "the animus . . . displayed against the women conductors on the omnibuses as they passed the procession," and the attempt by "a party of demonstrators" to drag "a young woman off a service car in which she was driving an officer who, by the way, did nothing to assist her." In 1920, an article in *Time and Tide* lamented the fact that as a result of the Great War "many people have become . . . mentally and morally unstable, and that in consequence crimes of a certain class are to-day alarmingly common over the entire country. Among these crimes is that of child outrage."[3]

Accounts of sexual attacks upon women filled the columns of newspapers. Gibbs reported that "the daily newspapers for many months have been filled with the record of dreadful crimes, of violence and passion. Most of them have been done by soldiers or ex-soldiers." He was struck by the

> brutality of passion, a murderous instinct, which have been manifested again and again in . . . riots and street rows and solitary crimes. These last are the worst because they are not inspired by a sense of injustice, however false, or any mob passion, but by homicidal mania and secret lust. The murders of young women, the outrages upon little girls, the violent robberies that have happened since the demobilizing of the armies have appalled decent-minded people.

The Vote, explaining "Why Carriages Reserved for Women are Needed," reported that "a young soldier, described in court as a desperate and dangerous man, was charged with assaulting a girl, aged 16, a domestic servant, in a railway carriage . . . . he sprang at her and caught her by the throat . . . . the accused said . . . he would have 'done her in.' "

Gibbs blamed "the seeds of insanity in the brains of men" on the "abnormal life of war" and on women who gave them venereal disease. In this version, the war and women become confused. "Sexually [the men] were starved," he argued.

> For months they lived out of the sight and presence of women. But they came back into villages or towns where they were tempted by any poor slut who winked at them and infected them with illness.

Men went to hospital with venereal disease in appalling numbers. Boys were ruined and poisoned for life.

The return of the soldier to a Britain in which women played a much larger role in politics and the economy than ever before was seen to pose a serious threat to the stability of the country, marked by disorder in virtually every realm of life—political, social, economic, and personal.

Political disorder appeared, for many, as a threatening consequence of the new franchise enacted in the 1918 Representation of the People Act, which established universal manhood suffrage and gave women over 30 the vote. The age requirement ensured that women would not enjoy a majority over men, whose numbers had been greatly reduced in the slaughter of war; fears of women "swamping" men at the polls loomed over the debate. Moreover, the age restriction ensured that those eligible to vote were likely to be wives and mothers; those excluded were largely single, unattached women who had made so significant a contribution to the war effort, who might seek to continue their work after the war and even to sacrifice marriage and motherhood to do so. The sexual disruption these women represented produced acute anxiety in the postwar years. The new electorate, comprised of newly emancipated women and, seemingly, of frightening, angry, out of work demobilized soldiers, alarmed a good part of society.

Conservatives, for whom property qualifications had served as guarantors of political responsibility, recognized that their traditional strategies would not survive the postwar political world of a mass electorate, necessitating the cultivation of a more broadly based constituency. They decided to continue the wartime coalition with Liberals and Labour, not believing that they could win an election on their own, and pursued an election strategy designed to thwart the emergence of Labour as a viable party. The Coalition government of David Lloyd George, a Liberal, and Andrew Bonar Law, a Conservative, issued letters of endorsement—derided as "coupons" by the opposition leader Herbert Asquith—to those Liberals and Conservatives deemed loyal to the government; the tactic worked, and the Coalition government was returned to power with a hefty majority. In the context of the Russian revolution of 1917 and an outbreak of strike activity at home, fear of bolshevism obsessed many MPs and government officials and a considerable portion of the press and the public. The Coalition government adopted in 1919 a series of inflationary policies designed to absorb returning soldiers into the work force, stimulating the short-lived postwar boom.[4]

Socially, Britain appeared to be a new world altogether. During the war, women had joined the workforce in unprecedented numbers, taking jobs as munitions workers, agricultural laborers, tram conductors, ambulance drivers, frontline nurses, and, finally, after the disasters of 1916, auxiliary soldiers. The dismantling of barriers between men's and women's work and the evident joy women experienced in their new roles fostered a blurring of distinctions that had helped to form traditional versions of gender identity. Mrs Alec-Tweedie, for example, rejoiced in the fact that by the events of the war, "women have become soldiers." Moreover, she predicted, it might not be long before "we may have to have women fighters too." In this context, it is not surprising that anxiety about the war frequently took shape as anxiety about sex, or was articulated in sexual terms; as the war effort worsened attacks on women, and especially on women's sexuality, increased. Women who labored in the munitions factories and served in the auxiliary forces excited adverse comment; many implied that their earnings came from working an "extra shift," by which they meant prostitution. Siegfried Sassoon's autobiographical Sherston told of his Aunt Evelyn complaining of "the disgracefully immoral way most of the young women were behaving while doing war work." Before they even reached France, members of the Women's Auxiliary Army Corps were accused of loose living and of corrupting the morals of "our poor lads." Making no distinction between prostitutes infected with venereal diseases on the one hand, and young girls or women infected with "khaki fever" on the other, Arthur Conan Doyle wrote to *The Times* in February 1917 of "vile women...who prey upon and poison our soldiers...these harpies carry off the lonely soldiers to their rooms...and finally inoculate them...with one of those diseases." A December 1917 letter to *The Times* referred to women as "sexual freelances" who "stalked through the land, vampires upon the nation's health, distributing and perpetuating among our young manhood diseases which institute a national calamity." In July 1918, Imperial War Conference attendees heard tales of infected women "lying in wait for clean young men who came to give their lives for their country." The government, for its part, introduced regulation 40d of the Defense of the Realm Act in March 1918, at the height of worries about the German advance, declaring that "no woman suffering from venereal disease shall have sexual intercourse with any member of His Majesty's Forces, or solicit or invite any member to have sexual intercourse with her." Clearly, in the minds of many Britons, sex presented as great a threat to the survival and existence of England as did Germany; the two were, indeed, conflated in the minds of many.

Mrs. Alec-Tweedie made this connection abundantly clear when she warned that "every woman who lets herself 'go' is as bad as a German spy, and a traitor, not only to her sex, but to her country."[5] These visions of sexuality in which women had become fully as unrestrained as men threatened traditional gender and sexual arrangements.

For many, the opportunity to contribute to national life, to work and to be well paid, was a rewarding and exhilarating experience, one that they would not easily have turned their backs on upon the conclusion of hostilities. The independence and autonomy they had found during the war could be construed as having been achieved at the expense of men, to whom they had no intention of relinquishing their freedoms. Rathbone's Joan noted that "men came back to homes which had been running perfectly well without them; to children whom they didn't know; to wives who had been free and well-off on separation allowances, and who resented having to submit once more to male interference, and to perpetual male presence."[6] Lady Rhondda recalled that

> we found ourselves in an utterly changed world. Across that gulf of chaos whose memory we needed above all else to wash away, the frontiers of 1914 were already dimmed and half forgotten. We could not, even had we wished, join this new comparatively sane world on to the jagged edges of the one that had broken off five years before—this new one was quite a different place. The war had broken down barriers and customs and conventions. It had left us curiously free.

She, like many other women, divorced her husband and proceeded to live a life of independence.[7]

Something like the blurring of gender lines that took place during the war continued afterwards, as young women of virtually every class— called, derisively, "flappers"—dressed in boyish fashions, cut their hair short, smoked cigarettes, drove cars, and generally pursued an active, adventurous lifestyle. Their counterparts, the "bright young things," men who had been too young to go to war in the years 1914–1918, offered themselves as effeminate contrasts, till it appeared, in the popular press at least, that young men and women had simply switched roles, characteristics, and styles with one another. Boyish women and effeminate men dominated the fashion pages of newspapers and magazines, representing the carefree, youth-oriented, pleasure-seeking, even hedonistic nature of the postwar generation sick and tired of a devastating war to which they had been unable to make a contribution; for others they constituted proof that society was in a complete state of disorder—disorder represented in gendered and sexualized terms.

The sexual disorders thrown up by the war and its immediate aftermath had to be managed, somehow, if normalcy and order were to be returned to postwar Britain and the men and women who served in the war reclaimed for the nation. One way to accomplish that aim involved creating a sexual peace between men and women by re-establishing a version of separate spheres for men and women.[8] But another way was to displace onto groups regarded as "borderline figures," "alien others," the impulses and instincts associated with sexual deviance and sexual disorder and then to eliminate those "others" from the imagined nation.[9] We see this process at work in the debates surrounding the passage of the Aliens' Restriction Act of 1919; the race riots in the port towns in 1919; British reactions to the mobilization of black troops in the Ruhr on the part of pacifists, socialists, and feminists in 1920; and the appeal of extreme right-wing politics—shading from Die-Hard conservatism into proto-fascism—for an important portion of the population.

The Aliens' Restriction Act of 1919 emerged as an outgrowth of the anti-German fervor that seized Britain in the summer and fall of 1918 and dominated the platform pledges of the "coupon election." Promises to "hang the Kaiser," to make the Germans pay for the war, and to expel all Germans from Britain responded to a broad-based xenophobia and Germanophobia that characterized Britain in the last months of the war. Although Lloyd George first tried to frame the issues of the election in terms of postwar recovery, he was compelled by pressure from politicians and the press on the radical right—Die-Hard MPs like William Joynson-Hicks, Kennedy Jones, Noel Pemberton Billing, Horatio Bottomley, and Henry Page Croft; the *National Review*, *John Bull* (later the *Vigilante*), the *London Times*, the *Morning Post*, the *Spectator*, and the *Daily Mail*—and from the electorate to sign on to the assurances of men like Bonar Law that "if this Government is returned to power at the conclusion of the peace, we shall send [interned Germans] back to their own country. We shall not only send back those whom we have interned, but we shall not allow others to take their places." In December 1918 Lloyd George declared that "it would lead to inevitable irritation and disturbances if Germans who had been fighting us for the last four years came over to this country to take the bread out of the mouths of the men whom they had for four years sought to destroy."[10]

Seeking to neutralize the radical right backbenchers in parliament, the Coalition government introduced a new Aliens' Restriction bill, seeking to extend the 1914 Aliens' Restriction Act, a simple enabling law giving the government emergency powers to issue Orders in Council pertaining to any alien whatsoever, not merely enemy ones. The Order in Council promulgated under the 1914 act empowered the Home Secretary to refuse entry and to deport any person in Britain whose presence he determined was harmful to the public. The 1919 bill rendered the 1914 act—intended for use as an emergency wartime measure—a peacetime provision by removing from the statute the language "at any time when a state of war exists between His Majesty and any foreign power, or when it appears that an occasion of imminent national danger or great emergency has arisen;" it would actually extend the powers of the Home Office.[11] Between April and November of 1919, parliament debated the terms of the Aliens Restriction bill: some opposed it because they regarded it as divisive and anti-Semitic; most opposed it because it did not go far enough to rid the country of "undesirables." It "is permissive in its character," complained Bottomley; it failed to serve as a "breakwater against the alien tide," the *Daily Mail* protested, to help create a "new 'Britain for the British.' "[12] Those who most vociferously raised their voices against aliens—members of the radical right—have been dismissed as being outside mainstream conservatism, but it is a measure of their influence both in and out of parliament that their concerns prevailed. In a move that surprised the government, the House of Commons defeated the initial bill by 185 votes and sent it back for strengthening. Led by Sir Edward Carson, the opposition included 120 Coalition Unionists and a significant number of Liberals and Labour trade unionists. The Home Secretary submitted a much stronger bill, which conferred upon him the authority to decide what nationality an alien held if there was some question about it. The act also made provocation of industrial disruption or sedition in the armed forces or among the civilian population subject to heavy penalties.[13] Participants in the debate over the bill initially identified as "enemy aliens" Germans or Austrians; very soon, however, they included "neutral" aliens, aliens in general, in their condemnation with no discrimination between the two. Indeed, MPs seemed eager to conflate them. As Bottomley said flatly, "every alien at this moment is prima facie an undesirable alien." "The enemy alien has been spoken about a good deal," intoned Sir Ernest Wild. "I am not sure the neutral alien is not as dangerous as the enemy one." Such statements introduced a "spirit of persecution," MP Colonel Wedgwood protested in the parliamentary debate, and eliminated at a stroke centuries of tradition of "assimilating this foreign element and teaching it that England is something worth living for." William Joynson-Hicks, who would become Home Secretary in Baldwin's cabinet in 1924, dismissed him and his concerns by declaring, in language we will revisit below, that Wedgwood is "a chartered libertine in this House," linking sexual promiscuity with tolerance of those who were not British.[14]

Aliens threatened the nation in a number of ways. Most concretely, in the aftermath of the Russian revolution, they were alleged to be responsible for the spate of strikes that had plagued the country since the armistice. MP Stanton, a longtime Welsh labour activist, denouncing "all the muck, the rubbish, and the refuse of the Continent and other places" that were "drift[ing] into this country," identified virtually all aliens as bolshevists and accused them of inciting workers to down tools. "We can well understand why there have been so many strikes and so much trouble and agitation," he declared. MP R. Carter echoed his charges, claiming that

> the unrest that at present is prevailing in this country has a very great deal to do, to my mind, with the alien enemy. You never hear of any disturbance, rioting, or anything of that kind without a fair sprinkling of aliens. Bolshevism, of course, is introduced in England almost entirely by aliens.

Pemberton Billing predicted that "if the alien agitator is allowed to take a hand in the game there will be bloodshed in this country in the next twelve months." Some MPs explicitly tied aliens to labour organizations, labour unions, and to the Labour party itself.[15]

"The whole object of this Amendment," asserted Sir Courtenay Warner, "is to exclude foreigners from having power to lead Labour organisations." Brigadier-General Henry Page Croft went further, tying the Labour politicians to

> Mr. Litvinoff, who was hailed by the whole of the Labour party as the ambassador of the new Republic of Russia. Mr. Ramsay MacDonald and his colleagues were very much upset that anything should be said derogatory to Mr. Litvinoff.... it was found that the Russian ambassador in that case was spreading revolutionary literature, that he was known by half-a-dozen names of various descriptions, that his real name was Finklestein, that twice he had been convicted of fraud.

This conflation of aliens with bolsheviks and then with Jews was a prominent and constant feature of the debates.[16]

A less concrete but no less powerful issue of the debates concerned keeping Britain for the British. Pemberton Billing declared, "I am deeply and sincerely anxious that the country should be reserved for our own countrymen and women." Joynson-Hicks argued for "the preservation of this country for the English people," while Mr R. McNeill went so far as to say that the determination "to keep our own country for our own people" far outweighed issues of housing, health, land acquisition, and reconstructive reform generally. "That was really the issue upon which this House was to a very large extent returned," he claimed.[17]

Opening Britain to foreigners, that is, to Jews, risked contaminating "all that is best in our national character." Disease, drug use, gambling, vice, and "unnatural offences," MPs insisted, endemic to "Asiatic" populations (using the term Asiatic in reference to Jews) would be brought into Britain and be allowed to flourish; and as "Asiatics" did not assimilate but kept to their own communities and preserved their own culture, they could not but act as "a source of weakness and danger" to the country. Sir H. Nield asserted that "these immigrants, in so far as they belong to the Jewish faith, do not assimilate or harmonise with the native race, but remain a solid and distinct community whose existence in great numbers in certain areas gravely interferes with the observance of the Christian position." Pemberton Billing announced that "I prefer my country to any other, and I want to see it preserved, and I want to see it saved from the Asiatic." Captain Ormsby-Gore's declamations against the "naked anti-Semitism" and "Jew-baiting" of Pemberton Billing did nothing to elevate the tone of the debate.[18]

"Aliens" represented sexual deviancy and sexual disorder. "All that is clean in the British character has been debased by the type of alien that has invaded us," Pemberton Billing lamented. "They have debased our morals in the lower standard, and they have debased our morals in the higher standard." Jews from Eastern Europe were believed responsible for the vice in the East End of London. "Vice!" sputtered Wild,

> why they are at the bottom of one-half, at least, of the vice of this Metropolis and of this country. The white slave traffic, unnatural vice, the exploitation of English girls whom they marry, and then live upon the proceeds of their prostitution; the brothel keepers who are too clever to be caught, because they keep in the background; the people with gambling hells [*sic*] who lead young men to destruction, and who bring in such horrible practices as doping and unnatural offences—that is the sort of atmosphere that has been introduced into this country by these people.[19]

The desire to establish firm, clear boundaries against foreign "others" became associated with fear of a different kind of otherness that threatened to breach the boundaries not only of the nation but also of the self—sexuality.

Most intangible, but most powerful, were the fears of aliens threatening to overwhelm the boundaries that safeguarded Britain's and Britons' very existence; references to breaches in the defenses of the country permeated the language employed by MPs to argue their positions. Britain would be "overrun with hordes" who "come in by the million;" this "tide of immigration" placed the country in "even greater danger of invasion than we were in 1914," announced Pemberton Billing. "The late Lord Chancellor quite recently stated that there were 20,000 aliens waiting in Holland ready to swarm into England directly the opportunity presented itself, and not only to swarm but to spawn." Aliens "sweeping down upon us," "pouring into the country," "flood[ing] our shores," had to be kept at bay at all costs.[20] The imagery conjured up in the 1919 debate contrasted markedly with that of the debate over the Aliens bill of 1905, in which language tended to be that of a controlled flow, of precision and order, of easy containment. Britain seemed possessed of clear, solid, defined boundaries for MPs in 1905. The flow of aliens was managed and directed; only once or twice did anyone mention "swamping." They "come to this country," said one MP who supported the restrictions, in language suggesting not hordes or floods of dangerous aliens but immigrants in measured amounts. Even the numbers used to support the provisions of the act in 1905 were precise and usually very small. "In 1900," declared one MP, "3,130 alien prisoners were received in our prisons, and in 1904 the number was 4,774." "In the year ending 31st March last no fewer than 308 such persons, who voluntarily admitted that they were either rejected in America or other countries abroad, arrived in the river Thames." "Recently 700 people of this character arrived in Liverpool." The 1905 bill targeted Jews, to be sure, but object of the 1905 bill was to control *undesirable aliens*, not all aliens. "It is the object of this Bill to draw a clear distinction between alien friends and alien enemies," explained Home Secretary McKenna, as the House debated the 1914 bill, differentiating quite finely between the two.[21]

The government used the extended powers conferred upon it by the 1919 act to close down the immigration of Jews to Britain and to deport many alien Jews, especially those in the East End of London. Certainly, this had the effect of creating hardship for and fear within the Jewish community there. But perhaps the most serious use of the powers of the state to restrict immigration and keep "Britain for the British" affected the black communities of the country, the term "black" referring to Indians, Asians, Arabs, Africans, and West Indians alike. Not content with restricting immigration, but unable to limit the freedom of black seamen under the terms of the 1919 act, Baldwin's government issued the Aliens Order of 1925, which made it possible for the state to deport even British subjects from its shores.[22]

This act derived in part from a series of race riots that rocked port towns in Britain between January and August of 1919, the likes of which, in terms of the widespread nature of the violence, were not seen again until the urban riots of 1981.[23] First in Glasgow and then in South Shields, Salford, London, Hull, Liverpool, Cardiff, Newport, and Barry, tens of thousands of white Britons, mostly male, set upon communities of blacks who had settled there. The riots produced a number of deaths, countless injuries, hundreds of arrests, and many thousands of pounds in property damage. The government responded to them initially by instituting a scheme of repatriation—the removal of black seamen to their countries of origin—and then by passing legislation that delineated all black seamen, whether subjects of the British crown or not, as "aliens."

Blacks had long maintained settlements in Britain, but up until 1914, their numbers had been small. The need for labor occasioned by the war expanded the black population—largely male—considerably. Present in virtually all wartime industries, their numbers were concentrated in the maritime forces, leading to a dramatic increase of black sailors and seamen in the port towns of Great Britain. The dearth of figures makes it impossible to estimate the number of black seamen who participated in the war, but of the 15,000 merchant seamen who lost their lives during the conflict, more than 3000 of them worked on what were called "Asiatic" contracts. When the war ended, blacks serving in non-maritime industries tended to gravitate to the port towns, where established interracial settlements of blacks and whites offered a hospitality not evident elsewhere in Britain.[24]

Violence directed against blacks by whites began first in Glasgow, in January, when some 30 Sierra Leonean sailors and firemen, all British subjects, were set upon by white seamen in the yard of the Mercantile Marine offices. Chased through the streets, they were finally rescued by local police, but not before one of them, Tom Johnson, was stabbed, and two white men, Duncan Cowar and Thomas Carlin, were shot and stabbed respectively. The Sierra Leoneans were thrown in jail, though charges against 27 of the 30 arrested were dismissed by the court.

One white man was arrested and found guilty of assault on a police officer.[25]

In South Shields the following month, a West Indian and nine Muslim sailors from Aden—all British subjects—were confronted by a large group of white seamen—British and foreign—and local white men at the Tyneside Shipping Office. A mêlée ensued, during which the crowd threw stones and bottles at the ten men. Over the next few days and sporadically into March, British and foreign whites and black seamen fought one another. In one instance, Abdulia Hassan was attacked by a group of British soldiers, who struck him and cut off his watch and chain with a knife. Hassan fought back, slashing one of the soldiers with a razor. As was true in Glasgow, and would be evident in the subsequent rioting, the black victims of the violence were cast as instigators and were arrested in numbers far outweighing those of their white attackers.[26]

Riots broke out in the East End of London in April 1919, and lasted through August. On 16 April, white seamen besieged a restaurant on Cable Street owned by an Arab, throwing bottles and bricks at the black seamen inside. Eight Muslims, one white seaman, and two policemen were injured in the fracas, though only Muslims were arrested for assault. In May, four days of full-scale rioting took place in the Limehouse area of the East End involving, according to some accounts, four to five thousand people. In this instance, crowds of whites attacked blacks with fists, stones, and knives. They laid siege to a boarding house where some 100 black men resided; as the *Eastern Post and City Chronicle* described it,

> a pitched battle . . . raged in the commercial Road between Limehouse Church and the Sailors' Palace for three hours. It culminated in a rout of the black men, who were driven into St. Ann's Street. The conflict continued until the police drew a cordon across the road to quell the riot.

In June, the Chinese community in Poplar came under attack; one house was "stormed" by a white crowd, its "furniture thrown out into the street and set on fire, while the occupants of the house were roughly treated, and one had to seek police protection . . . . There was some talk of wrecking the whole of the Chinese quarter," the *East End News* reported, "but the vigilance of the police prevented any such happening."[27]

In Salford and Hull, rioting against blacks broke out in early June 1919 and continued right into 1921. Beatings of black men and the vandalizing of houses inhabited by blacks characterized those riots, as was the case in Liverpool, which saw some of the most widespread rioting of 1919. Liverpool police finally gave up trying to control the violence against the black community, estimated to be some 5000 strong, ceding sections of the city to mob rule for three days. The Liverpool police reported that on June 9 and 10,

> a well organized gang consisting principally of youths and young men, soldiers and sailors, ages of most of them ranging from 18 to 30 years, . . . commenced savagely attacking, beating and stabbing every negro they could find in the street, and many of the negroes had to be removed under police escort to Gt. George Street Fire Station for their own safety. When no more negroes were seen in the street these gangs began to attack the negroes' houses . . . and in some cases they completely wrecked them.

One black man was "beaten severely about the head with the buckle end of a belt." Another, Charles Wooton, was chased by a crowd of whites to the dockside and forced into the water, where he drowned. Thomas Archer, a Jamaican who witnessed the event, testified to Trinidadian authorities that Wooton "was grabbed from the police by the dock workers who threw him into the sea and started to stone him whenever he came to the surface of the water until he was killed."[28]

In Newport, on 6 June, just hours after the *Monmouth Evening Post* reported the news of the Liverpool riots, rioting broke out in George Street, when a white soldier struck a black man over an alleged insult to a white woman. A crowd of whites

> surged around the corner to Commercial Road and smashed a restaurant owned by a Black man named Delgrada. From here the crowd moved on to Ruperra Street, where a Chinese laundry and an Arab boarding house were attacked. For two hours the rioters had everything their own way, it taking all that time for a body of police of suitable strength to appear on the scene.[29]

The most serious rioting took place in Cardiff, where over the space of four days in June three men lost their lives, dozens received wounds serious enough to require hospitalization, and the city sustained £3000 of damage to property. Police gained control of the white attacks on blacks in Cardiff by cordoning off Bute Town, the area of black settlement, from crowds of whites who sought to get through; with the assistance of troops, they prevented a situation that "would have been disastrous," noted the Cardiff Watch Committee, though disastrous to whom was startling. "If the crowd had overpowered the police and got through," the committee report claimed, "the Black population would have probably fought with desperation and inflicted great loss of life."[30]

Though they did not dominate the crowds involved in the rioting,[31] demobilized soldiers and sailors nevertheless figured prominently in the attacks on black seamen, a fact that should give us pause. They participated in and sometimes led the assaults in every city that saw racial violence that spring and summer. Contemporaries attributed their presence in part to the unemployment situation: returning from a war in which they had sacrificed so much to find their jobs filled. The *South Wales Evening Express* described "a house...being attacked by a crowd at the head of whom were Colonial soldiers." "The tone of the crowd was angry.... Several colonial soldiers present constituted themselves the ringleaders of the besieging party, which was largely made up of discharged soldiers. Some of the latter asked, 'Why should these coloured men be able to get work when it is refused to us?'" The *Liverpool Courier* told its readers that the riots had broken out owing to "the fact that large numbers of demobilised soldiers are unable to find work while the West Indian negroes, brought over to supply a labour shortage during the war, are able to 'swank' about in smart clothes on the proceeds of their industry."[32]

Some officials and members of the public justified the attacks on black seamen by alleging, contrary to the facts, that they had not done their part in the war. The *South Wales Evening Express and Evening Mail* told of a "Soldier Arrested" for assault on a black man. "The crowd demanded the soldier's release, and several persons cried out, 'He is one of us, and has fought for us, not like the blacks.'" The Chief Constable in Liverpool echoed these remarks when he wrote to the Ministry of Labour that the white men involved in the riots "took greater risks during the war than most of the coloured men, many of whom...stopped ashore to avoid the submarine menace." Men of color refused the portrayal of them as cowards and foreign parasites on the British host. Dr Rufus Fennel, heading a deputation of blacks to the Cardiff parliamentary committee, told the committee that "these men were not aliens, but British subjects, and had made sacrifices for this country." "The unprecedented spectacle of coloured men appealing to a British crowd for 'fair play' was witnessed in Hyde Park on Saturday," reported the *South Wales Evening Express*, quoting a speaker as telling the crowd, "men of colour are British to the backbone 'an if we were wanted again to-morrow to fight under the Union Jack not a man would hesitate.' "[33]

Where black seamen were perceived by the crowd to have fought in the war, they were treated leniently. The *South Wales Evening Express* noted that "a couple of the discharged British West Indies men have had the foresight to wear their uniforms when venturing abroad, and the sight of their badge has stood them in good stead." In "Coloured Man a War Hero," it reported on a black man who had been attacked,

> receiving several blows. For a while he took refuge in a shop, and the police ... were soon in attendance. While the man was under cover police quietly passed the word around that the refugee was an ex-soldier—a former member of the British West Indies Regiment. This had the desired effect, and the police were not interfered with as they escorted their man to a place of safety.

In another incident that reveals the public's association of war service with Britishness, the paper reported that "one of the coloured defendants had fought with the Monmouthshire Regiment in the war, and it was reported that he had taken sides with the white men during the recent disturbances."[34]

Along with unemployment and the insistence that priorities should be given to wartime service, newspapers, police officials, and court witnesses cited the resentment generated among the returning soldiers by the association of black men with white women, a theme that permeated accounts of and commentary about the riots in every instance save that of the first riot in Glasgow. The *Daily Herald*, indeed, neatly conflated the three issues in its 13 June 1919, story, quoting W. Sullivan of the National Sailors' and Firemen's Union as he asserted that

> the trouble is due to the refusal to ship the blacks who were imported in large numbers when our men were in the Army and Navy. All over the country officers ... hold that the white men who have done the fighting should be shipped before the blacks. They are actuated only by patriotic motives. There is nothing against the majority of the blacks .... the officers are firm .... They are saying: 'Men who have fought must have preference.'

Without pause or transition, Sullivan went on to assert that "the white girls in the East End—Poplar in particular—are fermenting trouble by their actions. The Home Office ought to step in." For many, in fact, the root cause of the race riots was the relationship of black men with white women. The *Herald* declared that "in all the places where trouble has arisen white women have in some measure been at the root of the disturbances." "Mr. Hobden [of the Seamen's Mission] agreed that sex contributed very largely to racial complications. White women are to some extent responsible, he said."[35]

The *Times* explained the riots in Liverpool as having been a consequence, in part, of interracial relationships.

> During the war the colony of coloured men in Liverpool, largely West Indians, increased until the men now number about 5,000. Many have married Liverpool women, and while it is admitted that some have made good husbands the intermarriage of black men and white women, not to mention other relationships, has excited much feeling.

In a letter to *The Times*, Ralph Williams justified the violence against black seamen on the grounds that miscegenation could not be tolerated. "Intimate association between black or coloured men and white women is a thing of horror," he declaimed. "It is an instinctive certainty that sexual relations between white women and coloured men revolt our very nature.... what blame... to those white men who, seeing these conditions and loathing them, resort to violence." The *Daily Chronicle* intimated that "the racial feud which has existed [in the East End of London] for some time past" arose from the mixing of white women with Chinese men. "In Northumberland-road, Poplar, a large crowd of people, including many soldiers, surrounded a house in which a Chinaman and a white woman were living. Both were forced to leave the premises, after which the mob ransacked the place." The *Times* recounted an incident in which,

> led by a soldier, several of the crowd, on entering a house in Hornfray-street, were confronted by a party of four white girls in night attire. 'We are British girls,' one of them said. 'Thank god there are others,' was the answer from one of the leaders, meaning that there were white girls who would not consort with black men. The four girls were hastily brushed aside and the house search for coloured men, but the search proved fruitless.

The reporter pointed out that

> some of the more sober-minded citizens of Cardiff consider that the coloured men are not alone to blame for the disturbances, although, at the same time, they deplore the familiar association between white women and negroes, which is a provocative cause. There are over a thousand coloured men out of work in Cardiff, most of them sailors, and it has to be remembered to their credit that during the war they faced the perils of the submarine campaign with all the gallantry of the British seaman. The negro is almost pathetically loyal to the British Empire and he is always proud to acclaim himself a Briton. His chief failing is his fondness for white women.[36]

Some of the allegations of miscegenation were linked to the fears expressed about "aliens"—read Jews, read bolsheviks—being raised in the debates over the 1919 Aliens' Restriction bill, which ran concurrently with the riots. The *Liverpool Courier* asserted that the race riots had been instigated by foreign enemies. In its 16 June 1919 issue, it referred to

> dangerous foreigners...plotting the break up and downfall of the British Empire.... They believe that if only they can stir up British men by showing up in the most disgusting fashion all intercourse between black men and white women, then they will be on a fair road to accomplishing their objects.

And just as aliens must be kept out of the country in order to keep it strong and pure, blacks should not be allowed to weaken the nation through their interaction with whites. The race riots offered "a lesson for England," declared the *Morning Post*: while whites could beneficially rule over blacks, whites and black could not live together in equality. "You cannot give full privileges as 'a man and a brother' to other racial types without accepting them also as brothers-in-law; and that path leads to racial degradation," the paper asserted.

> It is the sex question, indeed, that is the marrow of the matter. The coloured man so soon as he is treated as an equal aspires to be the mate of the white woman. That is the real test of equality for him, and it is a logical enough test. But all the instincts of the white race refuse that.

Faced with the realities of interracial settlement, the *Post* reassured readers, "Great Britain will now understand better the 'White Australia policy' and Western Canada's objection to unrestricted Asiatic immigration."

Local and national authorities appeared to share this conviction. Their immediate response was to separate the parties from one another. In Cardiff, the police forcibly confined blacks to the area around the docks known as Bute Town, where blacks had long settled, but beyond which they had recently expanded their residence. In Liverpool, the need to provide protection to many hundreds of members of the black community from white attackers by evacuating them from their homes and housing them in another part of the city led some to regard this as a potentially permanent solution. One correspondent to the Liverpool *Evening Express* urged the city to

> allocate these coloured men and their families to 'compounds.' Give each man a tally…and enforce him to be in his compound at a certain time…. This is the way the native is treated in Capetown, Johannesburg, etc., and, if any killing is done, it is usually one of his own race who is the victim.

The Lord Mayor and the Head Constable seemed to be thinking similarly; they met with a Ministry of Labour official to determine how best to deal with the black population in Liverpool. "In all probability," reported the Liverpool police, "the negroes will be accommodated in one or more of the camps which were occupied by troops during the war."[37]

The second response of local and national government leaders was to eliminate what they saw as the source of the problem. Contrary to the preponderance of evidence, police officials persisted in asserting that the riots had been instigated by blacks and called for the removal of black seamen from the port towns. "If the Government could repatriate the Black men without delay," wrote the Lord Mayor of Liverpool to the Colonial Office, "it would relieve the irritation which the presence of these men causes to our men." Indeed, the Liverpool riots stimulated the renewal of government repatriation efforts that had begun in February 1919 by the Board of Trade in response to high unemployment in the shipping industry. Originally directed at the black seamen who had come to Great Britain to help in the war effort, the repatriation scheme soon turned to all black seamen in the country, regardless of how long they had lived in their communities.[38]

Representatives from the Board of Trade, the Colonial Office, the Home Office, the Local Government Board, the India Office, the Ministry of Labour, and the Ministry of Shipping met in June to discuss how best to effect the repatriation of blacks, who had shown no inclination to leave the country. Repatriation committees were set up in the towns where rioting had taken place to assist the process: they were charged with collecting data about the "numbers, nationality and countries of origin of the coloured men in the port;" publicizing and explaining the repatriation schemes to "the coloured men;" helping "any coloured men who have a genuine claim to reside in this country" to find work; and advising them to accept repatriation "and point out the difficulties that they are likely to experience in obtaining work if they remain in this country." A resettlement allowance of £5, along with a voyage allowance of £1, it was believed, might encourage black seamen to sign up, though Viscount Milner, Secretary of the Colonial Office, offered a different rationale for the payment later in the month.

> I am seriously concerned at the continued disturbances due to racial ill-feeling against coloured men in our large sea ports. These riots are serious enough from the point of view of the maintenance of order in this country, but they are even more serious in regard to their possible effect in the colonies...when these men get back to their own colonies they might be tempted to revenge themselves on the white minorities there, unless we can do something to show that His Majesty's Government is not insensible to their complaints.... I am convinced that if we wish to get rid of the coloured population whose presence here is causing so much trouble we must pay the expense of doing so ourselves.

The refusal of a provision to include the white wives of black seamen in the scheme, however, proved to be sufficiently great an obstacle to the success of the program that the policy was overturned within months. Officials determined at a 30 July 1919 meeting of the interdepartmental group that "coloured men with white wives should not be repatriated for obvious reasons and that in so far as coloured men are married to other than white women, that these men would be repatriated with their wives." Fears of destabilizing race and gender norms in the empire by allowing miscegenation there stood at the heart of the policy to exclude white wives from the repatriation scheme. By 1 September, the repercussions of the policy became clear in the numbers of black men who refused to leave their families, and the policy changed.[39]

Finally, the officials discussed the possibility of interning black seamen while they awaited their return, as had been suggested by Liverpool
authorities. Minutes of the initial meeting recount the representative of
the Colonial Office asking "whether anything could be done in the way
of interning these people." The Home Office representative

> replied that if they were willing to be interned, it could be done;
> but although the War Office had placed a camp at Liverpool at the
> disposal of the local authorities for the purpose, when it came to be
> made available it was found that the men had gone back to their
> homes.

In the absence of voluntary internment, which seemed unlikely, the
Home Office was reluctant to impose any kind of mandatory confine-
ment on the black populations of British towns.[40]

Repatriation, despite the protestation of officials to the contrary, was
not a great success. Some 1200 black seamen left British ports between
July and September 1921 for the West Indies and the Mideast. The
limitations of the scheme compelled the government to utilize the provisions of the Aliens Restriction Act of 1919 and the Aliens Order of
1920 to effect their aims of eliminating blacks from Britain. Originally
aimed at restricting foreign immigration, especially that of Jews, the
order soon became the vehicle by which all blacks, whether or not they
were British subjects—and entitled to all the rights of British subjects—
could be refused entry to British shores. Invoking the powers invested in
him by the Aliens Order of 1920, Home Secretary Joynson-Hicks issued
the Coloured Alien Seamen Order in 1925; it required all "coloured"
seamen "who cannot produce documentary evidence of British nationality to register with the police as aliens," and to subject themselves to
fingerprinting. Home Office officials knew that few seamen, regardless
of race or nationality, carried passports. Instead, they relied upon their
"continuous discharge books" to establish their identity. In the case of
black seamen, even British black seamen, the discharge books would
no longer be accepted as proof of British nationality; for white seamen,
British or alien, it would still be accepted. "In the space of a few years,"
notes Laura Tabili,

> Black seamen went from welcome additions to the empire and partic-
> ularly to the seafaring workforce, with or without 'proper passports;'
> to undesirables denied entry to U.K. ports or deported when desti-
> tute, whether subjects or aliens; to presumptive aliens illegitimately

in Britain. At the same time the boundaries of the undesirable target group broadened... to all undocumented Black seafarers, including men the Home Office knew were British but could not prove it.[41]

As Barbara Bush has pointed out, "the perceived 'colour problem' related to very small numbers." Perhaps 5000 blacks, largely from West Africa, lived in Liverpool; in Cardiff, some 3000 black seamen resided, about two-thirds of whom were African or British subjects of African descent. The other port towns contained even fewer black seamen.[42] The wildly disproportionate response of Britons and the British government suggests that motives of a deeply psychological nature underlay the violence on the part of whites and the measures taken to remove blacks from British society. The near obsession with miscegenation bespeaks a profound concern about the maintenance of boundaries among returning soldiers and the public alike.

These fears of miscegenation found acute expression during 1920 when, in April of that year, France sent troops into Frankfurt, at the head of which was a company of Moroccan soldiers. Their presence, and that of the Senegalese "tirailleurs," set off a campaign, instigated by the Germans, to remove "black" troops from the occupation of the Rhine. The resulting furor took on international dimensions; in Britain, it was fomented by the publication in the *Daily Herald* of E.D. Morel's "Black Horror on the Rhine."

Morel was a prominent figure in British political life, associated with a variety of progressive causes pertaining to colonialism, disarmament, peace, and labor. He was supported in his campaign by a veritable *Who's Who* of labor, peace, and feminist activists: the Trades Union Congress, the Fabian Women's Group, Eleanor Rathbone of the National Union of Societies for Equal Citizenship, the *Women's Leader*, the Women's International League for Peace and Freedom, the Union of Democratic Control, the Women's Co-operative Guild, the National Federation of Women's Workers, the Federation of Women Teachers, the Association of Women Clerks and Secretaries, and the Standing Joint Committee of the Women's Industrial Associations. Within a month, Morel's pamphlet had sold 5000 copies, running to eight editions by April 1921.[43]

The language employed by all of those publicizing the use of black troops by the French burst with imagery of excesses of every kind. "FRANKFORT RUNS WITH BLOOD," screamed the *Daily Herald* on 9 April 1920. "FRENCH BLACK TROOPS USE MACHINE GUNS ON CIVILIANS."[44] The next day the paper declaimed the "SEXUAL HOR-ROR LET LOOSE BY FRANCE ON THE RHINE. DISAPPEARANCE OF

YOUNG GERMAN GIRLS." In the accompanying article, authored by Morel, readers heard, in frankly sexual imagery, that "France is thrusting her black savages still further into the heart of Germany." "There they have become a terror and a horror unimaginable to the countryside, raping women and girls," which, "for well-known physiological reasons," Morel explained, recalling centuries of lore regaling the sexual capacity of African men, "is nearly always accompanied by serious injury and not infrequently has fatal results."[45] The editorial page picked up the thread of the argument, urging its readers, "especially our women readers," to raise their voices against "the sexual outrages that are being committed."[46] Day after day for over two weeks, the *Herald* rehearsed the charges against the black troops, which it described in language to which we have become alert, as "an invading horde of savages:" "BRUTES IN FRENCH UNIFORM. DANGER TO GERMAN WOMEN FROM 30,000 BLACKS," despairing, again in revealing language, that "it is impossible to control the black levies."[47]

Morel's *The Horror on the Rhine*, published by the Union of Democratic Control in August 1920, fleshed out the points of his articles in the most scurrilous detail. For "races inhabiting the tropical and sub-tropical areas of Africa," he told his readers, "the sex-impulse is a more instinctive impulse, and precisely because it is so, a more spontaneous, fiercer, less controllable impulse than among European peoples hedged in by the complicated paraphernalia of convention and laws." Mobilizing African troops to occupy the Rhineland, given their "sexual requirements," necessitated that "in the absence of their own women-folk they *must be satisfied upon the bodies of white women.*"

> In ones and twos, sometimes in parties, big, stalwart men from warmer climes, armed with sword-bayonets or knives, sometimes with revolvers, living unnatural lives of restraint, their fierce passions hot within them, roam the countryside. Woe to the girl returning to her village home, or on the way to town with market produce, or at work alone hoeing in the fields. Dark forms come leaping out from the shadows of the trees, appear unexpectedly among the vines and grasses, rise from the corn where they have lain concealed. Then—panic-stricken flight which often availeth not.[48]

In partnership with the Women's International League of Peace and Freedom, the *Daily Herald* sponsored a protest meeting on 27 April 1920, in the Central Hall in Westminster. Morel's address reiterated all the claims and charges published in the past two weeks, but he added an ominous note. Using black troops to patrol German cities, with all the accompanying problems, he warned, would lead whites to "an intensification of fear, aggravating race prejudice, begetting harshness and cruelty." It would inculcate in blacks feelings of "contempt" and "loss of respect" for whites, it would destroy "a legend of superiority" whites enjoyed among blacks and would provoke among them the question: "Why, after all, do we suffer these people?" Raising an explicit possibility of annihilation, he declared that "wars of extermination between the two races" would ensue should race mixing continue.[49]

Other publications were a bit more circumspect. W.H. Dawson, in the *Contemporary Review*, decried "the scandalous employment of black troops, the admitted sexual excesses of these Africans...and the setting up of filthy French brothels in tranquil and clean little towns." His distress over disturbing the order of the towns rivals that over "sexual excesses,"[50] again suggesting fears of chaos and disintegration. *The Nation* protested against "the outrage of quartering semi-savages in the...midst" of Germany, calling their presence "an outrage on civilization."[51] The *Woman's Leader* initially condemned the use of black troops in fairly mild terms, calling it "a grave mistake," but four months later, when it looked as if the French were about to send black troops to Vienna, the paper reminded readers that "not six months ago white women all the world over were up in arms at the outrageous policy of quartering black troops in German towns, with its inevitable consequences."[52] For his part, Lloyd George believed the use of black troops in Germany so egregious that "we may have to repudiate our allies." What "if the Germans sent niggers from German Africa to Newcastle?" he demanded in a cabinet meeting. "Frankfurt is a proud city!" Once more associating fears of sexual excess with fears of annihilation, he told his colleagues, "people here would say we can only die once, we won't stand this insult."[53]

The same conflation of miscegenation, sexual excesses, and annihilation evinced by these accounts, but joined now to "the spectre of Bolshevism" found further expression in a review of books treating "the colour problem" by Frederick D. Lugard, former Governor-General of Nigeria. One of the books, *The Rising Tide of Colour*, by the American Lothrop Stoddard, raised the prospect of "a pan-Coloured alliance for the universal overthrow of the white hegemony at a single stroke, a nightmare of race-war beside which the late struggle in Europe would seem the veriest child's play," a possibility Lugard did not dispute. Encouraged by bolsheviks, who purportedly welcomed miscegenation as a means of bringing about communist revolution, "admixture with alien races" would bring about "the deterioration of the Nordic race-type" and ultimately annihilate the white races. "The union of opposite types, such as the Negro or Australoid with the Nordic," Lugard noted, ostensibly recounting Stoddard's thesis, "rapidly tends to the elimination of the latter, owing to the prepotency of the black race." As befitting a servant of empire, Lugard took the occasion of the review to pronounce "the true conception of the inter-relation of colour: complete uniformity in ideals, absolute equality in the paths of knowledge and culture, equal opportunity for those who strive, equal admiration for those who achieve," but, in the realm of the physical and the material, of the social and racial, "a separate path, each pursuing his own inherited traditions, preserving his own race-purity and race-pride." The danger of annihilation of whites through intermarriage with blacks necessitated the establishment of "drastic immigration laws." "Only by rigidly guarding his frontiers, and by restriction of immigration, can he preserve his race purity and save himself from extinction," Lugard asserted.[54]

The obsession with miscegenation, the violation of boundaries, and the need to establish barriers to stave off annihilation we have seen throughout these pages recall the accounts by German *freicorps* of their campaigns against communists and socialists in the years immediately following the war. The proto-fascist *freicorps* member, argues Klaus Theweleit in *Male Fantasies*, dreaded communism as a source of dissolution of self. Representing a disavowal of distinctions between what is mine and what is yours; an effacing of private possessions, whether material or psychic, in a terrifying, "promiscuous mingling," communism evoked the very terrors of being swamped, engulfed, and swallowed up posed by the working-class women who populated their writings, women who were virtually synonymous with prostitutes in the minds of the *freicorps*. Communism bespoke "the mass," an amorphous entity without boundaries or borders, into which one might sink and never come out again, in the same way that women announced the chaotic, unbounded, uncontrolled disorder of sexual desire and sexual excess. Both threatened the existence of the defined, definite individual self. In this rendering, the revolutionary communist mass and the flood are inseparable; given the language we have seen employed by Britons that conflates aliens with Jews with bolsheviks with blacks with sexuality, Theweleit's claim that "the *alien* race appears... to be the most intense embodiment of the terrors represented by the mass" becomes crucial to our understanding of the British campaigns against aliens and blacks in the early 1920s. The terrors of the mass could only be neutralized through the invocation of those traits that marked off Anglo-Saxon

Briton from black or Jew (and, as we shall see, Irish and Indian as well). In place of the messy, disorderly, chaotic impulses characterized by Jews and blacks, the Briton of the alien debates or the race riots posited himself as an individually—defined and—structured, autonomous part of a collectively—defined and—structured, autonomous whole. Maintenance of his own pure "race seems to protect him from disintegration," Theweleit argues. Miscegenation, the collapsing of borders separating one race from another, inferior one, on the other hand, "would inexorably cause him to disintegrate." Unable to distinguish boundaries that delineate self from other, fearful that the boundaries that establish the integrity of the self have given way before the onslaught of uncontrollable forces, the "soldier male" of the *freicorps*, and we need add, our very own Briton, cannot counter the threat of disintegration without resort to violence—linguistic or literal—against those forces that have so destabilized him.[55]

Theweleit's insights help us to understand in new ways the appeal of various fascist tendencies in the 1920s. Fascism was not simply a political ideology; indeed, that aspect held little appeal to Britons. It also held out the psychological and cultural promise of repair and wholeness. Britons turned to political movements that promised to shore up a precarious sense of a whole, coherent self, whether that be the individual self or the collective nation, political movements that, if not explicitly fascist in orientation, articulated many of the sentiments and performed much of the psychological work characteristic of fascism. In the past historians dismissed fascism in Britain as a foreign, insignificant movement, but within the past 20 years or so it has become evident that important segments of British society embraced certain aspects of fascist ideology with open arms. As one historian put it, "to suggest that there were any unique elements within British society which made it immune to the threat of fascism, is to illustrate an extraordinary complacency founded upon misplaced arrogance." In fact, asserts another, historians have underestimated the strength of fascist ideology and sentiment in Britain in the 1920s; the degree to which "fascist notions could find support and sustenance within British politics" was considerable. We have missed it because we have tended to examine it in terms of continental fascism—for which the genocide of National Socialism stands as the signifier—instead of placing it in the context of "mainstream politics or wider concepts of British culture." Certainly the anti-Semitic activities of the British Union of Fascists under the leadership of Sir Oswald Mosley have captured the attention of historians, but as Tony Kushner has argued, we should regard "the 1920s as an era of formative influence, one which, in some senses, influenced state policy on race issues far more than the 1930s."[56]

Fascism's promise to make the shattered subject whole again attracted a significant number of military and naval personnel of all ranks to a variety of organizations like the British Fascists (BF) in the 1920s. The level of participation of the armed forces prompted the Army Council in 1925 to proscribe membership in the British Fascists; the Navy announced in a Fleet Order that year that it was "undesirable" for active-duty sailors—though not reservists—to join the BF.[57] Some 60 percent of the leadership of fascist organizations had served in the armed forces; about 40 percent of them had fought in the Great War.[58] But fascist organizations enjoyed support from a broad array of society, from such mainstream publications as the *Morning Post* and the *National Review* and from "disgruntled and frustrated right-wing Conservatives," as Die-Hards like Joynson-Hicks, Brigadier-General Croft, and others prominent in the Aliens Act debates have been described.[59] Anti-Semitism, as we have seen, permeated those debates; but it proved to be a potent force outside of parliament as well. Most infamous was the campaign conducted by the *Morning Post* against Jews, who, the paper insisted, constituted the "overwhelming majority" of bolsheviks. In a series reproducing aspects of the forged "Protocols of the Elders of Zion," the paper laid out "the existence of a vast Pan-Oriental Conspiracy" to provoke "world unrest." It warned of the bolshevik tendencies of the labor unions, attributing the incidence of strikes to their infiltration by "International Revolutionaries" directed by "Lenin's Third International." Arguing that "the audacious threat of the miners" was thwarted only because organized labor as a whole was not yet "ready for revolution," the paper declared that revolutionaries were compelled to look elsewhere, to the empire, to Ireland and India, to continue their agitation. As we shall see in the following three chapters, the conviction that bolshevik revolutionaries were behind the rioting in the Punjab, the war for independence in Ireland, and the efforts by Labour to win a living wage was widespread and deeply held.[60]

Anti-Semitism was not new in 1919, to be sure, but it differed from its prewar incarnations: where it had appeared largely as a "cultural prejudice" before 1914, now it had become, in the hands of disillusioned right-wing individuals, factions, newspapers, and journals, "a conscious ingredient of British political life." It found expression among far many more people than those sympathetic to fascist or proto-fascist groups. *The Times*, for instance, ran a series of articles entitled "Alien London" in October and November 1924, two years after "an intense but transient burst of anti-Semitism during the years from 1918 to 1922" was said to have come to an end.[61] Published in the aftermath of the election that put Labour out of office and re-instated a Conservative government, the articles told of the "swarms" of "strangely picturesque Hebrew characters which one instinctively associates with astrologers, magicians, and other mysterious people." Living in "inconceivable filth and squalor," these immigrants from Poland or Ukraine are "naturally alive to the eloquence of the 'Red' gospel." Having driven out the native British and the respectable, anglicized Jews from the neighborhoods in the East End, "they do not form a desirable element in our population, and still less a desirable element in our electorate . . . . These people remain an alien element in our land."

"The invaders" have "degraded the local standard of living in many quarters;" the youth among them, who "are physically more precocious than the British," engage in "immorality" to such an extent that the age of puberty among "British children in some areas" has been lowered. "The Jew, also, is notoriously a sufferer from nervous disorders. Hysteria is frequent among the immigrants, and during the air raids large numbers of them displayed a shocking and dangerous lack of self-control which was a byword among Londoners." British Jews, by contrast, demonstrated far less "excitability and nervousness," presumably having been steadied by exposure to native British behavior and expectations. "Alien Jews" in the East End not only panicked during air raids, they "did their best to avoid military service." Again, by contrast, "a large proportion of the British-born children of aliens followed the fine example set by the British Jews, and played their part like men during the war." The series stood as an apologia for the use of aliens restrictions to deport undesirable Jews and to keep out others who sought to make London their home. Denying that anti-Semitism drove anti-alien legislation, *The Times* protested that having lost so many men in the war, Britain could not afford to admit "prolific aliens," many of whom had been "exposed to the wildest revolutionary influences."[62] The distinctions drawn by *The Times* between alien and British Jews— a distinction invoked by many Anglo-Jews themselves—was not shared by Die-Hards, as we shall see in the next chapter.

Talk of the pernicious effect of "aliens" on British social, economic, political, and cultural life had permeated the election campaign of 1924. One of the main factors in Labour's loss was the publication of the Zinoviev letter, which purported to prove communist influence within Labour party circles, but an equally important element in that "exceptionally dirty campaign" was the anti-alien rhetoric infusing the speeches of Conservative politicians. Stanley Baldwin, portrayed as a man of moderation, morality, and reconciliation, opened the door for the more vociferous of his anti-alien colleagues in a speech broadcast on 16 October 1924, in which he told listeners that alien subversives had been behind the domestic unrest of the country. "We cannot afford the luxury of academic socialists or revolutionary agitation," he warned his countrymen, and declared, "I think it's high time somebody said to Russia 'Hands off England.' "[63] As Prime Minister, Baldwin appointed to the Home Office William Joynson-Hicks, a man he knew would vigorously enforce the policies of the 1919 Aliens Restriction Act. In the first days of his tenure, a delegation from the National Citizens Union, a right-wing group that had considered merging with the British Fascists when he, Joynson-Hicks, was its vice-president, lobbied him to pursue and expel the aliens who so degraded British society. He promised to use his powers of deportation liberally, a vow he kept throughout the five years he held office. He based his decisions to naturalize aliens or not on "whether the applicant has, so far as can be judged, become an Englishman at heart and has completely identified himself with English interests."[64] Those he found wanting could expect no quarter; he expelled hundreds of non-naturalized Jews, many of them Russians, for violations under the Aliens Act. He refused, as he put it, to "see England flooded with the whole of the alien refuse from every country in the world."[65]

Joynson-Hicks' appointment as Home Secretary, which historian Ross McKibbin characterizes as "in retrospect almost unbelievable," should alert us to broader tendencies within the Conservative party. For while he has been regarded as a figure of fun by contemporaries and observers of the period alike, his anti-alien, anti-bolshevik, anti-Semitic sentiments were in deadly earnest, sentiments shared by mainstream conservatism. Joynson-Hicks heard no "dissent against his activity from within the government, least of all from the bucolic, tranquil Baldwin." His biographer demonstrates that he was, in fact, a popular member of his party who was willing to say what his colleagues thought, and we should regard his cabinet appointment not as "a sacrifice of good sense to the Tory right," as one historian puts it, but as "a desirable representative of elemental Toryism." In fact, fascism's relative weakness in Britain derived from "the inability of the Fascist movement to attract large numbers of right-wing Conservatives away from their 'natural' party." The Conservative party offered the same kind of answers and solutions to the problems thrown up by the war. "Britain's strong

Conservative Party," notes one historian, "virtually monopolised the ground on which any fascist movement might hope to base itself."[66]

Fears of "social disintegration" in consequence of the enlarged electorate and of gains made by workers during the war obsessed those who might have, in the absence of the Conservative party, turned to fascist programs. The unity and strength of the nation, they worried, might well dissolve in the face of threats from within and without. "Aliens"— Jewish and bolshevik—were behind all of the forces that sought to destroy the "British way of life." Conservatism, like fascism, promised to shore up the country, to unify society through the mobilization of certain "integrating myths," as G.C. Webber calls them. He sees the invocation of those myths—categorized under the notions of ruralism, religion, and cultural renaissance—as "deliberate attempts to revive the philosophy of nineteenth-century toryism,"[67] a body of thought, I would argue, entirely unequipped to deal with the shattered subject of the postwar period. Rather, the narration of "integrating myths" that took up the entirety of the 1920s involved struggles over the composition of the "nation" itself. Who could be said to belong to the nation? This question was resolved following a series of incidents and developments that progressively narrowed the framework within which a whole, coherent, sturdy, unified national identity could be established. As those who did not meet the criteria were extruded (Jews, West Indians, Indians, Irish, Africans) or re-fashioned (workers, women), a "nation" capable of performing the ideological work necessary to heal the shattered psyche of postwar Britons and of weathering the storms of the 1930s was forged.

3
The Amritsar Massacre, 1919–1920

For me the battlefield of France or Amritsar is the same.
To this day women hush their children with the name of
General Dyer.[1]

On 13 April 1919, Brigadier-General Reginald Dyer ordered a patrol of
Indian troops under his command to fire on a crowd of some 25,000
unarmed Indian men, women, and children in the Jallianwallah Bagh
in Amritsar. About ten minutes later, their ammunition virtually spent,
he ordered them to cease shooting. Hundreds of people lay dead, thousands more wounded littered the ground. Dyer led his troops from the
Bagh, leaving the injured to fend for themselves; the curfew imposed
on Amritsar kept would-be rescuers from collecting the dead and getting medical attention for the wounded until the next day. Many died
overnight.

The Amritsar massacre, as it came to be called, provoked a crisis in
British and Indian affairs. For Indian nationalists, it marked the moment
at which home rule within the empire would no longer be enough;
nothing less than independence would do and the "Quit India" movement took off. For Britons in India and at home, it set off a heated
controversy about the nature of British rule—about the nature of Britishness itself. Emotions ran high as issues of the greatest importance were
debated, revealing a nation profoundly disturbed about the direction it
would take in the aftermath of the Great War.

The Amritsar massacre offers us a window on the workings-out of
trauma on both the individual and the collective level. Dyer's explanations for his behavior and the justifications offered by his defenders

64

betray massive anxieties about their ability to maintain psychic wholeness in the face of an onslaught of terrifying forces—"hundreds of thousands of fanatical natives," as Commander Bellairs put it,[2] with all the threats of racial, political, and sexual contamination they conjured. These anxieties in turn compelled a nation-wide argument about British identity. The massacre should be seen as a consequence of traumas arising from the war, but it was also productive of trauma in and of itself, which would become manifest in subsequent colonial and domestic clashes over the next ten years.

The massacre at Jallianwallah Bagh followed a series of developments and events in India that resulted in widespread rioting across the subcontinent. In 1917, the Secretary of State for India, Edwin Montagu, had told the House of Commons that the government sought to gradually expand self-government in India by increasing the numbers of Indians in every part of the administration. One aspect of the reforms proposed by Montagu and the Viceroy of India, Lord Chelmsford, entailed giving greater representation to Indians in provincial assemblies, a prospect that generated a great deal of resistance among members of the Indian Civil Service (ICS) and the provincial governors, chief amongst them Sir Michael O'Dwyer, Governor of the Punjab. O'Dwyer and his colleagues insisted that the reforms would exacerbate the protests and rioting that had broken out in many provinces.

Conditions in the Punjab following the war made life difficult for a broad strata of the Indian population. Wages in industries that had prospered in wartime fell dramatically, catapulting much of the population into debt. The influenza epidemic had struck the Punjab particularly hard, taking up to 25 percent of the population in some villages.[3] Impoverished Punjabis often expressed their distress through protests, creating disorder throughout the province. The Defence of India Act, which had enabled the government to deal harshly with protestors during the war, had lapsed; colonial officials sought and received exceptional new powers to deal with disorder in the Rowlatt Acts, legislation that enabled the Viceroy to suspend due process of law and to imprison Indians without trial. The Rowlatt Acts inflamed Indian public opinion. The goodwill evoked by the Montagu-Chelmsford reforms vanished, replaced by anger, disappointment, suspicion, and mistrust. Educated Indians of all political stripes submerged their differences and united against the Rowlatt Acts under Mohandas Gandhi's *satyagraha* movement. Demonstrations took place in a number of cities, and rioting broke out in Ahmedabad, Delhi, and a number of Punjab provinces, prompting Lord Meston, an old India hand, to denounce "the new orgy of abuse and calumny" instigated by the acts. *The Times* utilized much the same imagery in its disgust with "the intolerable orgy of disorder arising out of the agitation against the Rowlatt Acts."[4]

Unaccustomed to seeing Muslims and Hindus, nationalists and loyalists, conservatives and liberals working together in concert, British officials jumped to an erroneous conclusion: that a revolutionary conspiracy, probably hatched in Moscow, sought to overthrow British rule and establish Indian independence. This conspiracy did not, in fact, exist, but fear of it informed the decision-making and actions of colonial and military officials, leading to severe repression against public processions and any other manifestation of protest. When, on 30 March and 6 April 1919, a series of peaceful *hartals*—a kind of religious general strike—shut down much of the Punjab, rumors of mutinies and plots to end British rule swept through the Anglo-Indian population. Believing themselves to be at risk for assault and murder, British officials and civilians began to arm themselves.[5]

In Amritsar, Deputy Commissioner Miles Irving ordered the arrest and deportation of two local leaders, Drs. Satyapal and Kitchlew, who, he believed, planned to incite the townspeople to violence. On 10 April, word of their deportation spread throughout the city, and, in concert with news of Gandhi's arrest in Palwal the previous day, spurred large crowds of Indians—unarmed—to congregate in the city center and make their way to the Civil Lines, the boundary separating the Indian from the Anglo-Indian population, in order to protest the arrests outside Irving's bungalow. Along the way, no violence occurred and no Europeans were assaulted. Upon their arrival at the bridges that crossed over the Civil Lines, however, the crowd met resistance from British troops, one of whom may have fired a shot without orders; when demonstrators tried to continue forward and took to throwing stones at the troops, they were fired upon. Official accounts put the Indian dead at 12, the wounded at 20–30. The shooting set off a day of rioting resulting in sabotage, looting, arson, assault, and the deaths by beating of five European men. Protesters cut telegraph and telephone lines and damaged the railways. Anglo-Indian women and children were hurried off to the fort, but not before Marcella Sherwood, the manager of the City Mission School, was badly beaten and left for dead in the street. Rescued and hidden by Hindu shopkeepers until they could get her to safety, she lay near death for days.[6]

That night, 10 April, the Commissioner of Lahore, A.J.W. Kitchin, arrived in Amritsar, took control from Deputy Commissioner Irving, and proceeded, in the words of one historian, with "what was to be a continual goading of the military to take violent measures against the populace." Kitchin urged the military commander from Lahore, Major MacDonald, to use "all military force" to check any further demonstrations and telegraphed O'Dwyer in Lahore of his intention "to prohibit and break up such processions with military force." O'Dwyer responded the next day with his approval and a promise to provide airplanes and armored cars. Kitchin began to plan with Irving to march troops through the city, "firing on every one they saw," according to the wife of the principal of Khalsa College, Gerard Wathen, who heard of their intentions. Wathen desperately tried to persuade Kitchin and Irving to give warning before firing, as the crowds of the night before had already dispersed and many hundreds of innocent onlookers and families seeking to bury their dead were out and about. Kitchin and Irving agreed to give warning, through Indian lawyers and professors from Khalsa, that all Indians must be off the streets and all burials completed by 2:00 P.M. "If at that hour there were any meetings or crowds they would be immediately fired on," reported Mrs Wathen. "At 2 aeroplanes were to ascend and if the crowds still persisted bombs were to be dropt." Major MacDonald, who voiced his objections to the ineffectiveness of the warnings and to any interference with funerals by the military, was replaced at Kitchin's insistence by Lieutenant-Colonel Morgan, who, presumably, could be counted on to be more aggressive in his dealings with Indians.[7]

At this point, the record becomes a bit confused. At 2:00 P.M., General Dyer claimed in his report, just as the funerals were taking place, he received orders to proceed to Amritsar and take command. Dyer's biographer, Nigel Collett, found no such order or mention of it in any of the relevant logs, and doubted that the order was issued at all. "It looks," he stated, "very much as though Dyer made his own decision to move to Amritsar, and that he sought to conceal this later."[8] The general arrived late the night of 11 April and immediately took charge.

No violence had occurred on 11 April, and the peace held on the 12th as well, by which time the Amritsar garrison had been strengthened and the "ringleaders" of the riots of the 10th arrested. Dyer made no effort to place his troops around the city to extend his control and preserve the peace, a decision reflective not of his competence but of his attitude toward Amritsar and its residents. His mission, he believed, was not simply to restore the city to order and re-establish civil authority; having declared war on the British, as Dyer saw it, Amritsar was enemy territory. "Something equivalent to a state of war existed between him and the people of the Punjab," noted the Marquess of Crewe in 1920.

"He speaks of the crowd at the Jallianwallah Bagh as the rival army." The whole area must be subjected to British rule and its citizens—enemy combatants—punished.[9]

On the morning of 13 April, Dyer, accompanied by Deputy Commissioner Irving and the Superintendent of Police, made his way through the city to issue a proclamation designed to quash any insurrectionary activity. At 19 different spots he announced his arrival with the beating of a drum and had read out in Urdu and in Punjabi the following:

> The inhabitants of Amritsar are warned by means of this proclamation that if they damage any property or commit any act of violence in the neighborhood of Amritsar, such acts will be considered to have been instigated from the city of Amritsar, and we shall arrange to punish the inhabitants of Amritsar in accordance with military law. All meetings and assemblies are prohibited by this proclamation, and we shall act in accordance with the military law in order to disperse all such assemblies forthwith.[10]

A second proclamation prohibited travel outside the city without a pass, established an 8:00 P.M. curfew, and banned any and all processions. Violations of these orders might be met with force of arms.

Shortly after noontime, Dyer was informed that a meeting would be held that afternoon in the Jallianwallah Bagh, a large enclosed plot of land in the center of the city. Neither Dyer nor Irving made any attempt to keep the meeting from taking place; they forebore to station any police at the entrances of the Bagh to prevent people from entering or to demand that those already there leave, and posted none of the proclamation notices they had made just hours earlier throughout other parts of the city. Instead, Dyer seized what appeared to him to be a golden opportunity to act. As his wife, Annie, stated later,

> How was he to fight the rebels, how was he to bring them to decisive action in the narrow streets and winding lanes of Amritsar? It was a problem ... which seemed to him, with his little force, insoluble, unless, indeed, he could get them somehow in the open. And that seemed too much to hope for .... But this unexpected gift of fortune, this unhoped for defiance, this concentration of the rebels in an open space—it gave him such an opportunity as he could not have devised. It separated the guilty from the innocent, it placed them where he would have wished them to be—within reach of his sword.[11]

Dyer planned carefully, choosing for his force 90 men who would not be loath to fire on Punjabis: Gurkhas, Baluchis, and Pathans, who hailed from territories beyond India's borders. He took no British soldiers, and opted to lead the force himself rather than delegate authority to the officers of the men he chose. As his biographer observes, "By dismissing these middle-ranking officers, Dyer ensured that there would be no officers present who might baulk at his plans. His choice of both commander and troops argues for the deliberate nature of what was to follow."[12]

With his special force and two armored cars, Dyer proceeded to the Jallianwallah Bagh just after 4:00 P.M. Upon his arrival, according to official accounts, he

> marched his infantry through a narrow lane into the Bagh and deployed them immediately right and left of the entrance. The armoured cars he left outside, as the lane was too narrow to admit them. Having deployed his troops Brigadier-General Dyer at once gave orders to open fire and continued a controlled fire on the dense crowd facing him in the enclosure...for some 10 minutes until his ammunition supply was at the point of exhaustion. 1,650 rounds of .303 mark VI ammunition were fired. The fatal casualties as the result of this action are believed to be 379; the number wounded has not been exactly ascertained, but is estimated...at possibly three times the number of deaths. Immediately after giving orders to cease fire, Brigadier-General Dyer marched his troops back to Ram Bagh.

None of the estimated 20,000 people assembled in the Jallianwallah Bagh had firearms, though some of them "may have been carrying sticks."[13]

Though he initially claimed that he fired on the crowd out of fear that his troops would be overwhelmed, Dyer later changed his story, and stuck with it till the end of his days. He had fired, he said in the later version, because the crowd had assembled in defiance of his orders in the proclamation. He continued to fire in order "to produce a moral effect in the Punjab."

> I fired and continued to fire until the crowd dispersed, and I consider this is the least amount of firing which would produce the necessary moral and widespread effect it was my duty to produce if I was to justify my action. If more troops had been at hand the casualties would have been greater in proportion. *It was no longer a question of*

merely dispersing the crowd, [italics in original] but one of producing a sufficient moral effect from a military point of view not only on those who were present, but more especially throughout the Punjab. There could be no question of undue severity.

He testified that "I had made up my mind that I would do all men to death if they were going to continue the meeting." Though the crowd had begun to disperse before he ordered his troops to open fire, he instructed them to continue, because, he explained, though "I could disperse them for some time; then they would all come back and laugh at me, and I considered I would be making myself a fool." He directed his troops to turn their guns on "places where the crowd was thickest." Had he been able to get his armored cars into the walled enclosure, he admitted, he would have used the machine guns mounted on them against the crowd, producing a much greater casualty rate. When asked if he had made any provision for the wounded, he told the commission,

No, certainly not. It was not my job. But the hospitals were open and the medical officers were there. The wounded had only to apply for help. But they did not do this because they themselves would be taken in custody for being in the assembly. I was ready to help them if they applied.

He failed to mention that the 8:00 P.M. curfew established two days earlier, violation of which could cause one to be fired upon by troops or police, kept Indians indoors that night, unable to collect the dead or get the wounded to hospital.[14]

One eyewitness watched the massacre from a house overlooking the Jallianwallah Bagh. "I saw hundreds of persons killed on the spot," testified Lala Girdhari Lal before the Congress party's inquiry into the events.

The worst part of the whole thing was that firing was directed towards the gates through which the people were running out. There were small outlets, 4 or 5 in all, and bullets actually rained over the people at all these gates.... many got trampled under the feet of the rushing crowds and thus lost their lives. Blood was pouring in profusion. Even those who lay flat on the ground were shot.... No arrangements were made by the authorities to look after the dead or wounded.... I then gave water to the wounded and rendered such assistance as was possible.... I went round the whole place and saw almost every body lying there. There were heaps of them at different places.... The dead bodies were of grown up people and young boys also. Some had their heads cut open, others had eyes shot, and nose, chest, arms, or legs shattered...I think there must have been over 1,000 dead bodies in the garden then...I saw people were hurrying up and many had to leave their dead and wounded, because they were afraid of being fired upon again after 8 p.m. [the curfew set on the 11th]...Many amongst the wounded, who managed to run from the garden, succumbed to injuries on the way and lay dead in the streets.[15]

The next day, Dyer met with a number of Indian notables to explain the situation to them. They were to open the shops, he declared, or be shot.

You people know well that I am a soldier and a military man, you want war or peace? And if you wish for war, the Government is prepared for war. And if you want peace, then obey my orders, and open all your shops, else I will shoot. For me the battlefield of France or Amritsar is the same.[16]

Given the powers of martial law on 15 April, which were backdated in order to encompass the violence of 10–13 April, Dyer proceeded to impose a series of punishments calculated to humiliate and debase the Indian population of Amritsar, the vast majority of whom had broken no law. He insisted that all Indians *salaam* to any Anglo-Indian he or she encountered. By the "crawling order" issued on 19 April, right after he had visited Marcella Sherwood in recovery, of which more later, he required any Indian passing through the lane where she had been attacked to go down on their bellies and crawl through the dirt and muck. "It is not suggested that the assailants of Miss Sherwood were the residents of the street," noted the Minority Report issued by the Hunter Commission, charged with investigating the massacre. "This order must have had the immediate result of seriously inconveniencing the residents of houses abutting on the street, and thereby punishing people who were *prima facie* innocent."[17] Contemporary photographs show soldiers of the 25th Londons, who had been invalided out from France in March of 1918, using their bayonets to prod a man on his belly along the "crawling lane."

Dyer also had erected there a triangle, or whipping post, on which six boys, unconvicted of any crime but suspected of beating Sherwood, were flogged. As one witness, a municipal employee, reported to the Congress party inquiry,

Sundar Singh was the first to be fastened to the flogging post (*tiktiki*) and given thirty stripes. He became senseless after the fourth stripe, but when some water was poured into his mouth by a soldier, he regained consciousness; he was again subjected to flogging. He lost consciousness for a second time, but the flogging never ceased till he was given thirty stripes. He was taken off the flogging post, bleeding and quite unconscious. Mela was the second to be tied to the post. He too became unconscious after receiving four or five stripes. He was given some water, and the flogging continued. Mangtu was the third victim. He too got thirty stripes. While Mangtu was being flogged, I cried bitterly, and as I could not bear the sight any longer, I lost my consciousness. When I recovered my consciousness, I saw the six boys who had just received flogging, were bleeding badly. They were all handcuffed, and, as they could not walk even a few paces, they were dragged away by the Police. They were then taken to the Fort.

Deputy Commissioner Irving regarded these extraordinary punishments as the means by which Anglo-Indian rage might be answered and assuaged. "The feeling among Europeans was desperately bitter," he claimed, "some civilians in the fort were saying what they would do to Indians when they got out, and I was seriously afraid of acts of reprisal." Dyer told O'Dwyer the same thing, substituting for bitter Europeans his British troops, who, he claimed, having witnessed the savage assault of English ladies and the murder of fellow countrymen, could barely be controlled. The punishments were intended to "make an impression" on them. This justification—that carrying out extraordinary punishments that were proscribed under civil law were necessary in order to contain the violence of British civilians and soldiers—would be resorted to later in regard to reprisals by Black and Tans in Ireland.[18]

Dyer's actions in Amritsar were approved by his immediate military and civilian superiors in the days following the massacre, though O'Dwyer felt it necessary to rescind the crawling order. When news of what had occurred reached the Indian government, however, alarm bells sounded. Chelmsford informed Montagu, who appointed a commission headed by Lord Hunter to investigate the circumstances of the shootings and the punishments meted out under martial law. After months of testimony, the Hunter Commission found that Dyer's actions merited sanction; the Government of India removed him from his position, and the Army Council recommended that he be retired from service, a recommendation the government accepted. A variety of interest groups mobilized against the government's actions, initiating a series of debates in the Commons and the Lords, in the columns of all the major newspapers and journals, and ultimately in the court of King's Bench, which vindicated Dyer. Support for Dyer was deep and wide. Most of the Anglo-Indian community; a large minority of MPs in the Commons; a majority of the Lords; and a significant number of private individuals who gave tens of thousands of pounds to the Dyer fund established by the *Morning Post* came to his aid. Most of the letters in the press approved Dyer's actions, while the Oxford Union could muster only a 130–121 vote in favor of the government's decision to retire him.[19]

What could have led Dyer to behave as he did, to shoot down an unarmed crowd of people, many of whom were sitting on the ground? By all accounts, except for Dyer's initial one, which he later changed, the crowd was peaceable: Sargeant Anderson reported that "I wasn't afraid. I saw nothing to be afraid of. I'd no fear that the crowd would come at us." Was it that Dyer was "insane," "an excitable lunatic of a man," as Lieutenant-Colonel Villiers-Stuart claimed in 1917, after serving under Dyer's command in India? During the war, which he spent in Persia, Dyer led reckless and violent attacks on clans that failed to support the British war effort, disobeying orders in doing so. Chelmsford told King George in 1920 that Dyer's wartime activities had given rise to the story "that to this day women hush their children with the name of General Dyer much as the Saracenic women used to frighten their crying babies with the name of Richard Coeur de Lion." But throughout the firing at Jallianwallah Bagh, reported Sargeant Anderson, "Dyer seemed quite calm and rational," though others found it impossible to display the same *sang froid* in the face of such bloodshed. At one point Dyer's adjutant, Captain Briggs, "was drawing his face up as if in pain, and was plucking at the General's elbow," as if to get him to stay the order. Two police officials accompanying Dyer's party, Superintendent Rehill and Inspector Jowahar Lal, found the situation intolerable, and left the Jallianwallah Bagh before the shooting ended. Rehill, asserted Collett, was so undone by the experience that he "denied having seen anything at all," a common response of traumatized individuals. But he later told his niece that he felt responsible for the massacre, and suffering from horrendous nightmares, turned to drink, "ending as a shadow of the man he had been." Dyer, for his part, never budged from his conviction that what he had done was right and proper. He may not have been quite sane, but he was entirely in command of his actions that evening in the Jallianwallah Bagh and in the days that followed.[20]

It seems that Dyer acted as he did in order to maintain his emotional equilibrium, to stave off unbearable anxieties about being overwhelmed by a mass of Indian people, no matter how peaceful they might be. In his written report to the General Staff of the 16th Indian Division dated 25 August 1919, Dyer noted that "we cannot be very brave unless we be possessed of a greater fear." As Collett has observed, such an admission in a military report was extraordinary. "It came from the depths of his soul," he argued. "Dyer's conception of his duty arose from his fears. He had killed, and would forever believe he was justified in killing, to allay them." Dyer knew that the crowd he faced at Jallianwallah Bagh was unarmed; and, he told the Hunter Commission, he believed he could have dispersed it without firing. It posed no threat to him at the time and, given the strength of the garrison in Amritsar by 12 April, could constitute no real danger to the city even were it to break out and take to the streets with violence. Dyer feared not the actual circumstances present in the Bagh that afternoon, but what that peaceful assembly of Indians represented to him: a threat to his physical and, more frightening, his psychic integrity. As he told a reporter for the *Daily Mail* upon his return to England, were he to have held back, "I and my little force would have been swept away like chaff, and then what would have happened?"[21] Like insubstantial and insignificant bits of waste, they might be blown away into nothingness.

Dyer and his supporters expressed these fears in images of flooding, of swamping, of breaching of defenses by an unstoppable force capable of sweeping away all in its path. This trope appeared in virtually every account of the events leading up to and culminating in the massacre at Jallianwallah Bagh, testifying to the agonizing concerns about maintaining boundaries and personal integrity characteristic of postwar Europeans. In these depictions, the "crowd" and the "mob" were not comprised of discrete and distinguishable individuals in large numbers but existed as an undifferentiated mass; the people involved in the violence of 10 April could not be separated out, in the minds of Dyer or his defenders, from those congregating at the Jallianwallah Bagh on the 13th; rebellion in the Punjab could not be kept distinct from rebellion everywhere. Indians took on the aspect of a globalizing entity capable of destroying individual Britons and the very empire itself. (The Marquess of Crewe, however, would not buy the argument, countering that Dyer's claim "that if he had not taken the action he did, that crowd, within a short space of time, would have destroyed all Europeans and all his troops...seems a hardly tenable statement,"[22] and injecting a little reality into a debate filled with fantastic imaginings of an unstoppable, engulfing force.)

Described variously as "a seething mob," a "vast sea of Indian humanity," "hordes from the city," "a wild crowd," "a furious crowd," "an absolutely mad crowd, spitting with rage and swearing and throwing stones," this mass of "fanatical natives" behaved in uncontrollable ways and its actions threatened to overwhelm the boundaries that established Britons as autonomous, discrete individuals. It *"burst over* Hall bridge," which connected the city to the Civil Lines, on 10 April. It *"swept through* the city on that terrible afternoon, ... calling for 'white blood.' " It *"came streaming out* of three gates towards the civil lines." It *"poured out* of the three gates ... it *surged* towards the civil lines," it *"swarmed* into the railway goods yard," it moved "like an approaching *flood."* At the Jallianwallah Bagh "the vast crowd which had been squatting on its heels seemed to *rise in a wave and subside and rise again." "Waves* of the panic-stricken *rushing* into culs-de-sacs [*sic*] *rushed back* again, and disappeared as they found an exit." Sir Edward Carson, in a House of Commons debate on 8 July 1920, insisted that Dyer's action "may have been that which saved the most bloody outrage in that country, which might have *deluged* the place with the loss of thousands of lives." The Marquess of Salisbury declared that "the authority of the Crown would have had to be reasserted in *rivers* of blood, if rebellion had once *burst* forth (italics added)."[23]

Dyer's defenders at the time and later repeatedly contrasted the size of his troops with that of the crowd, highlighting their fears of being overcome by an all-consuming but unrecognizable and unknowable threat. At Jallianwalla Bagh was "a crowd so big that had it rushed the little force it could have destroyed it, either with *lathis* or with naked hands," claimed a Dyer apologist. The *Morning Post* explained Dyer's actions by insisting that "with his tiny force audacity was his best hope, and he evidently resolved to strike a blow which would not only quieten Amritsar but settle Northern India;" he was "commanding a force so small that only by swift and resolute action could he hope for safety," it had asserted a few days earlier. "The mere rush of the crowd would have swept that slender force off its feet," argued Viscount Finlay, while Lord Ampthill allowed that "this very tiny force" led Dyer to believe he would have been "enveloped" by the crowd. Dyer's force was "so small," maintained the Earl of Middleton, that "the mere weight of the crowd would have annihilated it." In a letter to the *Spectator* retired Major-General J.E. Waller argued that "had he hesitated ever so little, he and his small force would have been annihilated."[24] The imagery of annihilation by an overwhelming force permeated virtually every account of the massacre.

The language used to represent the dangers of Amritsar reveals a broad swathe of Britons deeply worried about staving off threats of dissolution and annihiliation. The endless references to the vulnerability of

Dyer's tiny force at the hands of a massive crowd reveal an inability to distinguish the crowd at the Bagh from the rebel elements many Britons believed were at work throughout the subcontinent and else-where across the globe. In the face of evidence to the contrary, both Lord Finlay and Joynson-Hicks, for example, insisted, in a bid to demonstrate the warlike nature of the crowd, that no women or children had been present at Jallianwallah Bagh. Rather, asserted Finlay, "the people were there in multitudes. It was an assembly of men, many of them crimi-nals of the worst type, who had been engaged in the excesses" of 10 April, when, the *Morning Post* reminded its readers, "a great mob, many thousand strong, was surging into the civil lines."[25]

"Does any one doubt," demanded Lord Ampthill,

> that if General Dyer had done less, that this vast defiant mob of rebels would have dispersed to perhaps ten different places in order to resume the work of murder, pillage and arson, which they had commenced on the previous days. His object, and his right object, was to deter them from their murderous work.

"If you are dealing with a formidable mob," declared Lord Finlay,

> assembled in defiance of the express orders of the government, and at a time when an insurrectionary movement is in progress through-out the whole district, are you not justified, when you choose your way of putting down that insurrectionary movement, in doing it in a way which will have a beneficial effect on the restoration of order throughout the whole district? Where you have a state of things such as, unfortunately, existed in the Punjab (which really approximated to a state of war) strength is sometimes the truest mercy.

After all, the *Morning Post* exclaimed, "the whole of Northern India was in a seething agitation." "His object was to disperse, not merely the meeting in the Jallianwala Bagh, but the storm of rebellion that was hourly gathering over the length and breadth of the Punjab," it reminded readers. "For some days there was a very real danger of the entire European population being massacred," wrote an "English-woman" to *Blackwood's Magazine*. "General Dyer's action alone saved them."[26]

Above all, the specter of India in rebellion raised fears of violation of English women, a conflation of political and sexual outbreak given voice by countless commentators. As the *Morning Post* put it, "we may be certain that evil and dangerous passions smoulder under the ashes of revolt." The paper carried a letter from "A Briton" claiming that

> inflammatory and criminal posters were being persistently exhibited at Lyallpur calling upon the mob in the name of the blessed Mahatma Gandhi to outrage European women. 'What time are you waiting for now?' demanded these posters. 'There are many ladies here to dishonour.' And the rioters were incited to 'go all round India, clear the country of the ladies and these sinful creatures.' . . . The criminal manifestoes spread broadcast in Lyallpur give some idea of what might have been expected had the mob gained the upper hand.

A story in the same issue repeated these charges of incitement to rape Englishwomen to explain to its readers that

> one other consideration . . . may have been present to General Dyer's mind, . . . which, though not a pleasant subject to dwell upon, cannot be passed over . . . . The hideous possibilities that the idea opens up do not need to be enlarged upon. The isolation and defencelessness of Englishwomen in India makes them only too easy a prey.

Claiming that "such atrocities as those foreshadowed in the Lyallpur proclamations would arouse feelings that would never be satisfied with legal retaliation," the paper suggested approvingly that Dyer resorted to "the stern example in the Jallianwallah [*sic*] Bagh" in order to satisfy a vengeful blood lust that could not be appeased through legal means of prosecution and punishment. The paper hailed the fact that "the name of General Dyer is universally held in honour at the present moment by Englishwomen in Northern India who know what the situation was, though they cannot talk of it."[27]

Dyer, having spent his formative years in India, had been raised on the tales of the Indian Mutiny of 1857, stories of horror, however unfounded, that still gripped the Anglo-Indian population over 60 years later. Images of white women being raped and mutilated by Indian mutineers were never far below the surface for virtually all Anglo-Indians and could be readily conjured up. In fact, when riots broke out in Delhi in March, Dyer had been on a holiday driving tour with his wife and niece. They were set upon by stone-throwing demonstrators as they crossed the Sutlej river and someone pushed a log in front of the car, forcing

the driver to swerve to avoid a wreck. Unhurt, though shaken, they proceeded on, but Dyer, noted Collett, was greatly disturbed by the assault
on his wife and niece. The memory of the assault, he stated, "seems to
have underlain much of his thinking over the next few weeks." Indeed,
it was after visiting Marcella Sherwood, who was still in very serious condition, "swathed in bandages and lying between life and death," that he
issued the "crawling order" and had the six boys flogged in the "crawling lane." As he explained in his report to the General Staff and later
told the Hunter Commission, "a helpless woman had been mercilessly
beaten, in a most cruel manner, by a lot of dastardly cowards. She was
beaten with sticks and shoes, and knocked down six times in the street."
"It seemed intolerable to me that some suitable punishment could not
be meted out," he asserted. "Civil law was at an end and I searched my
brain for some military punishment to meet the case. Shooting was, in
my opinion, far too mild a punishment and it was for me to show that
woman must be looked upon as sacred."[28]

Prospects of violated white women obsessed the supporters of General
Dyer. Michael O'Dwyer wrote to the *Daily Telegraph* and *Morning Post* on
9 June 1920 that "General Dyer's action at Amritsar on 13 April smashed
the rebellion at its source, and *thus* [my emphasis] prevented widespread
bloodshed, rapine, and the murder of Europeans in the Punjab and
probably elsewhere." "Your Lordships will recollect that there were
many women and children who had taken refuge in the so-called fort,"
asserted Lord Finlay, "who, if the mob had triumphed, would have been
at their mercy. I shall not picture what their fate might have been." Even
Lord Buckmaster, who defended the government's decision to retire
Dyer on the grounds that he shot for too long in the Bagh, sought to
explain the general's actions by arguing that "an Englishwoman had
been assaulted and left for dead on the pavements of Amritsar. Proclamations had been issued that only thinly disguised an invitation not
only to personal violence against men, but to cases of dishonour against
women. General Dyer may well have thought that there was only a thin
white line that stood between the handful of European people . . . and all
the savage fury of a crowd who were maddened with seditious rhetoric,
and drunk with the new wine that ferments throughout the world,"
equating, again, sexual with political upheaval.[29]

The Right Reverend A.E.J. Kenealy, retired Roman Catholic Archbishop of Simla, wrote to the *Morning Post* that failure of the military
in India to act against "an anti-white man movement of so menacing
and widespread a character . . . would have meant the general murder of
European men, the outraging of women, the loot of public buildings

and the desecration of Christian churches." He warned, in what Collett described as "an oblique reference to the expected sexual assault upon European women," that "an Oriental mob has peculiar proclivities." To other audiences, he was not so oblique: he told Army Chief of Staff Sir Henry Wilson that "if we threw [Dyer] out we should lose India with untold murders and rape and chaos." For Kenealy, as for so many Britons, "oriental proclivities" excited meanings of despotism and sexual licentiousness, images of men in thrall to sensuality and pleasure who held their women in the worst kind of sexual slavery, providing a foil against which Britons could imagine themselves to be: manly men who held their women in awe and treated them with respect. The rape of white women by Indian men held particular terrors for Britons, for it suggested their inability to uphold the distinctions between Indian and Briton, threatening to extinguish masculine identity itself. Markers of British manliness, the purity of white women had to be protected and/or avenged if masculine identity was to be sustained. The *Post* carried a letter from E.P. Henderson, ICS retired, articulating precisely this concern: "O'Dwyer and Dyer, being *men*, met the trouble and broke it.... The streets of Amritsar, by the way, were placarded with posters urging the rape of all white women!" Had they not broken the trouble, preventing the not incidental sexual violation of white women, they would not be men, the letter intimated.[30]

Anglo-Indian women had no doubt about their fate at the hands of Indian rebels, having heard from birth the stories of the mutiny and internalized the prejudices about Indians expressed by their parents. When Dyer left India in April 1920, some 100 or so English women from the Punjab thanked him personally, assuring him that "we, who would have suffered most had the outbreak spread, are not unmindful of what we owe you." The *Woman's Leader*, official paper of the National Union of Societies for Equal Citizenship, formerly the National Union of Societies for Women's Suffrage, carried a letter from 679 English memsahibs, women "who know India, and the risk to the lives and honour of English women in time of rebellion, or even of serious local disorder." They wished readers to remember

> the treatment of Miss Sherwood at the hands of the mob, together with the actual attempts of the same mob to murder other English women, and the hardships inflicted on those who, with their children, were driven to take refuge in Amritsar fort and other places, as well as the placards posted at Lyallpur inciting to dishonour Englishwomen there.

The danger posed to English women equaled that of the worst times, they asserted:

> English women have never since the great Mutiny of 1857 been in such peril as they were in India in the spring of 1919, nor since the almost forgotten tragedy of Cawnpore, have Indian mobs, armed with dangerous *lathis*, been directly incited to the murder and outrage of English women, as they were in India last year.[31]

These fears of the violation of English women were not new; the constant invocations of the Indian Mutiny recall the countless—mostly groundless—tales of the rape and torture of English women at the hands of Indian rebels that circulated throughout mid-Victorian Britain in the aftermath of the Mutiny. But the imagery used by Dyer and his supporters to depict the events leading up to the massacre at Jallianwallah Bagh differed dramatically from the representations used to describe the events of 1857, reflecting a different kind of felt danger. Instead of masses, surges, waves, and other undifferentiated masses of people, the mutineers of 1857 formed themselves in organized, coherent, discrete, delineated units of force. They were not "hordes" or "vast seas of Indian humanity" or "seething crowds;" they were the "600 followers of Nana," the "50 Sowars," the "500 Nujeebs," the "4,000 mutinous troops," "an army of 25,000 men with 36 guns." Sometimes, indeed, they might be "a host well armed" seeking to "carry...the entrenchment by storm," but they acted in entirely recognizable and knowable ways. They did not "surge," they "set off" on orderly marches to the west; they did not "flood," they "returned to Cawnpore and halted...and took up a position;" they did not "pour out" or "swamp," they "attacked," "entered the place," "then proceeded to the intrenchments." They certainly killed Britons, whom they spectacularly outnumbered; they committed atrocities; they constituted a significant challenge to Britain's hold on India; but they did not appear, in the accounts of participants or subsequent reporters, to threaten personal psychic dissolution or annihilation. Anglo-Indians feared them, but in a manner consonant with prevailing models of subjectivity at the time: they could see the enemy, count them, strategize against them, handle them, and, ultimately, believed they could defeat them. They, in turn, committed atrocities against civilian Indians, but they did not confuse civilians with mutineers, as they did at Amritsar.[32]

The massacre at Jallianwallah Bagh provoked intense, even agonizing debate about the nature of British rule. On 8 July 1920, Sir Edward

Carson introduced in the House of Commons a motion to reduce the salary of the Secretary of State for India as a vehicle for expressing disapproval of the government's retirement of Dyer. The motion failed by a vote of 230–129, but only because Labour and Independent Liberal MPs voted with the Coalition government. Many Coalition MPs refrained from voting, an indication of the strength of support for Dyer. Two weeks later, the Lords took up the motion of Lord Finlay that "this House deplores the conduct of the case of General Dyer as unjust to that officer and as establishing a precedent dangerous to the preservation of order in the face of rebellion." This motion passed by a vote of 129–86.[33]

Montagu set the terms of the debate, presenting to the Commons two stark choices to those who would hold empire. "Are you going to keep your hold upon India by terrorism, racial humiliation and subordination, and frightfulness," he asked,

> or are you going to rest it upon the goodwill...of the people of your Indian Empire? There is no other choice—to hold India by the sword, to recognise terrorism as part of your weapon, as part of your armament, to guard British honour and British life with callousness about Indian honour and Indian life...[or to] ensur[e]...that order is enforced in accordance with the canons of modern love of liberty in the British democracy.

"Is your theory of domination or rule in India the ascendancy of one race over another, of domination and subordination," he asked his colleagues, "or is your theory that of partnership?" Dyer's supporters chose the former; they regarded the rightful dynamics of empire as those in which one race was, indeed, ascendant over and dominated a subordinate one, and argued that using force against elements bent on the destruction of the British in India was wholly justified. "Every country in the Empire is held by the sword," reasoned Lord Harris. "Whether it is Londonderry, or Dublin, or London, or India, we have eventually to come back to force to secure obedience to the law." Brigadier General Surtees wondered that there could be any

> member of this House who believes that we govern India with the approval of those governed by us? If a *plebiscite* were taken to-morrow as to who should govern India the result would be against us. If we do not hold India by moral suasion then we must hold it by force—possibly thinly veiled, but still by force.

Dyer had done what he had to do to maintain order and stability in the face of what was believed to be a conspiracy to overthrow British rule, he had upheld the very principles upon which empire had been won and was sustained. To think otherwise, to suggest that Indians might be allowed to join in partnership with Britons was to court danger, "as force is the only thing that an Asiatic has any respect for," as a Brigadier-General of the Delhi garrison told the Hunter Commission.[34]

This had been demonstrated beyond all possible doubt, insisted Dyer apologists, by the rioting following the introduction of the Montagu-Chelmsford reforms, which had led ultimately to the showdown in Amritsar. "Every element of sedition, every lawless and bloodthirsty instinct, encouraged by Mr. Montagu's reforms, smouldered into flame," editorialized the *Morning Post*. "Instead of censuring the gallant soldier whose action possibly saved the white inhabitants and loyal Indians from frightful carnage," blustered Henry Page Croft, "surely our bounden duty is to censure the man who created the situation which General Dyer was called in to save." Dyer had not been wrong, this line of argument went, Montagu had; to punish the wrong man and to do so summarily was to violate British principles of justice, fairness, and the rule of law. Edward Carson protested that Dyer had been treated unfairly by the Government of India and the Army Council. "You talk of the great principles of liberty which you have laid down," he argued in the House of Commons debate.

> General Dyer has a right to be brought within those principles of liberty. He has no right to be broken on the *ipse dixit* of any Commission or Committee, however great, unless he has been fairly tried—and he has not been tried.... I say to break a man under the circumstances of this case is un-English,

declaimed the Irishman. The Earl of Middleton announced his support for Finlay's motion on the grounds that the Government of India's "administration of justice" as it was brought against Dyer "has been imperfect" in its failure to act "as the one just force umpiring between all sections, races, nationalities, and creeds." Lord Ampthill declared that "for every man who may agree...that the treatment of the rebellious crowd at Amritsar was the grossest outrage in our history, there are at least a hundred who consider that the real outrage has been the treatment of General Dyer by the Imperial Government and the Government of India," a formulation in which the deaths of and injuries to thousands of Indians were trumped by the cashiering of a brigadier general. And the *Morning Post* wrote in an editorial, "Englishmen will tolerate a great deal, but they will not stand flagrant injustice. Nor will they acquiesce in Oriental methods of punishment without trial."[35]

This last comment about oriental methods of punishment was directed straight at Edwin Montagu, whom Brigadier-General Surtees referred to as "a right hon. Gentleman, sitting in Oriental aloofness in Whitehall." As a Liberal, Montagu might be regarded by Conservatives as an awkward member of the Coalition government, in which they held the preponderance of power; as a Jew, he was regarded by a significant portion of public opinion as an alien within the nation. Jews in government, for many Britons, served in ways antithetical to British interests. "Oriental," of course, was also used to characterize south Asians, placing Montagu squarely in the camp of Gandhi and his followers. In asserting that Montagu was not suitable for his office, R. Gwynne argued in the Commons that "his sympathies have been with those who are opposed to law and order in India, whilst he has been prejudiced against those who have been trying to maintain it." "If he is Mr. Gandhi's friend, he has no right to be Secretary of State for India." For Dyer's supporters, Montagu's Jewishness—what one writer called his "orientation," in a play on "orientalism"—explained, paradoxically, both his despotic treatment of Dyer and his advocacy of Indian self-government and friendship with Gandhi.[36]

The debate over Amritsar referred frequently to concerns about exciting "racial feeling;" though meant to refer to Indian sentiment, as often as not the term was as readily applied to Montagu as to south Asians. J.L. Maffey, the Viceroy's Secretary, wrote to Chelmsford about the debate in the House: to the "old 'true-blue' service section" that had "rallied in force" on behalf of Dyer, he recounted, "the only issues were: (a) Is it English to break a man who tried to do his duty? (b) Is a British General to be downed at the bidding of a crooked Jew?" During Montagu's speech, he was interrupted several times by cries of "Bolshevism!" Sir William Sutherland told Lloyd George that as Montagu warmed to his subject, he became "more Yiddish in screaming tone and gesture, and a strong anti-Jewish sentiment was shown by shouts and excitement among normally placid Tories," who, he feared, may have been riled enough to come to blows against the Secretary of State. Austen Chamberlain, the Chancellor of the Exchequer, lamented Montagu's apparent inability to read his audience, to appreciate the sympathy MPs had for Dyer whether or not they sanctioned his actions. "Our party has always disliked and distrusted him," he conceded, but Montagu's throwing down of the gauntlet guaranteed a violent reception. "On this occasion all their English and racial feeling was stirred to a passionate display—I think I have never seen the House so fiercely angry—and he threw fuel on the flames. A Jew, rounding on an Englishman and throwing him to the wolves—that was the feeling," he declared.[37]

The *Morning Post* informed readers that

> in Mr. Montagu's disastrous oration appeared the Oriental, pro-foundly imbued with racial bitterness, suffering torments, habitu-ally concealed, from the morbid delusion that he belongs to 'an oppressed people,' and solely inspired in all his Indian dealings with the fanatic motive of proving that an alien race is as good as the English.

"It was not the academic and obsequious Radical which stood forth, but the Oriental zealot," the paper declared, denouncing "the Orien-tal methods pursued by a Secretary of State who is resolved to free an 'oppressed' race from its 'oppressors,' while taking his salary from the said oppressors." The *Morning Post* began its fund drive on behalf of General Dyer on 10 July 1920, under the heading "These Be Thy Gods, O Israel." Two days later, on 12 July 1920, it began its serialization of "The Protocols of the Elders of Zion" under the heading, "The Cause of World Unrest (The Jews)".[38]

On 13 July 1920, the *Post* began to insinuate that Montagu's British-ness was suspect. He is "strangely ignorant of the psychology of the British people," the paper scoffed. "He did not understand—how should he?—that the British people love justice and fair-play." The next day, it went further, indignant that "the British instinct" for generosity towards its public servants "has been affronted—an instinct which is neither native nor familiar to Mr. Montagu."[39] Even for Dyer's opponents, Mon-tagu's House speech had demonstrated a marked indifference to British sensibilities, a lapse attributed to the traits characteristic of his race. *The Times*, which condemned Dyer's actions, castigated Montagu for his fail-ure to present the case against him in a measured, even, reasonable way. "Mr Montagu," it pointed out, "patriotic and sincere English Liberal as he is, is also a Jew, and in excitement has the mental idiom of the East." As a Jew, he could not be expected to appreciate "our inductive English method of political argument." Chelmsford echoed this view in a letter to Maffey, noting that any other orator would have been able to tune his speech to the ear of the audience he was addressing. He doubted this would be possible in the case "when the audience is Western and the speaker is Eastern." The debates over Dyer's actions in

Amritsar had raised the question of who could be counted as British.
For Dyer's supporters and for many of those who were not, the answer
was clear-cut: not Indians and not Jews, no matter how assimilated they
might be.

The Amritsar massacre and the debate it set off compelled the retelling
of a narrative that could incorporate the breaches that the behavior
of Dyer and the justifications of his supporters created in the story of
Britishness that had been fashioned as a part of the Great War. Britons
had undergone the most terrible of sacrifices in a war they fought
to defend the weak and to preserve democracy at home and abroad.
They had made promises of self-government to India in return for
substantial aid of the war effort. With Amritsar, many of them found
their ideals made hollow and their promises empty. Not only had the
country not lived up to its ideals, it had behaved in ways reminiscent of the enemy only recently defeated—Germany—and one which
now loomed large in the popular imagination, the bolsheviks. As the
members of the Hunter Commission who issued the Minority Report,
Sir C.H. Setalvad, Pandit Jagat Narayan, and Sahib-zada Sultan Ahmed
Khan, stated, in adopting "an inhuman...method of dealing with subjects of His Majesty the King-Emperor" Dyer had engaged in decidedly
"un-British" behavior. They likened his actions to that of the Germans
during the invasion of Belgium in 1914—"Prussianism," they asserted,
best characterized Dyer's thinking. At home, Britons insisted that Dyer's
behavior was unprecedented in the history of the country and of the
empire, an anomaly that had to be disavowed if the precepts of Britishness as they understood them could be upheld and possession of empire
vindicated.[40]

"Prussianism" found expression in the "terrorism" and "frightfulness"
perpetrated by Dyer in his determination to fire on the crowd at Jallianwallah Bagh until he could fire no longer so to make a larger impression
on the Punjab as a whole. "That is the doctrine of terrorism," charged
Edwin Montagu, and it could not be tolerated if Britain was to act in
its own best interests. Winston Churchill agreed. In "these anxious and
dangerous times," he pleaded,

> there is surely one general prohibition we can make. I mean a
> prohibition against what is called 'frightfulness.' What I mean by
> frightfulness is the inflicting of great slaughter or massacre upon
> a particular crowd of people, with the intention of terrorising not
> merely the rest of the crowd, but the whole district or the whole
> country.

He likened Dyer's actions to precisely "the bloody and devastating terrorism" he detested in bolshevism, contrasting it with "the august and venerable structure of the British Empire, where lawful authority descends from hand to hand and generation after generation.... Such ideas" as Dyer's actions represented "are absolutely foreign to the British way of doing things." Though in complete sympathy with those who feared "the general drift of the world's affairs at the present time" towards revolution, he could not countenance the methods they condoned in order to battle it. "This is not the British way of doing business," he insisted. "I shall be told that it 'saved India.' I do not believe it for a moment. The British power in India does not stand on such foundations. It stands on much stronger foundations." Lieutenant-General Sir Aylmer Hunter-Weston despaired that Dyer had called into question the army "as a national institution, which has the confidence and approbation of all right-thinking citizens." He worried lest "it should ever be looked upon as a menace to well-ordered civil liberty." "To allow anything in the nature of Prussian 'frightfulness' is entirely abhorrent to the British nation, and, therefore, to the British Army."[41]

"Fair dealing and humanity and justice to a weaker people," noted Lord Meston, had been the traditions governing the British empire, which Dyer's actions had "broken." He urged the Lords to show that "you do not endorse acts of violence; that you have an outlook higher than mere racial prestige." Lord Curzon, Secretary of State for Foreign Affairs, agreed, adding that "national honour" had been debased by the acts of "horror," "even of shame" endorsed by Dyer's supporters. Lord Carmichael, former Governor of Bengal, mused that "it may be necessary to shoot people sitting; I do not know," but he refused to believe that any Englishman, Scotsman, or Irishman, or any one belonging to the free countries within the British Empire, "approves of the feeling that lies at the basis of the 'Crawling Order.' " "Such a course of conduct...cannot be defended," declared Lord Birkenhead, the Lord Chancellor, in the House of Lords. "This has never, so far as my knowledge of the history of this Empire extends, been approached in all our long, anxious and entirely honourable dealings with native populations." Lloyd George's *Daily Chronicle* editorialized in support of the anti-Dyer faction, upholding "the broad principles, that the British Empire should rest on justice, and not on 'Prussianism.' " It disavowed the statements of those who would see Dyer as a heroic figure in a long and venerated tradition of British rule in India, arguing instead that the Amritsar massacre was "in direct conflict with all the principles to which the modern British Empire owes its existence."[42]

A number of prominent Britons scrambled to distance the country from the atrocities of Amritsar by bracketing the incident off from all previous and, presumably, all future governance of the empire and portraying the massacre as an anomalous, isolated aberration. Churchill, who, as Secretary of State for War, had brought the Army Council around to firing Dyer, characterized his actions as

> without precedent or parallel in the modern history of the British Empire. It is an event of an entirely different order from any of those tragic occurrences which take place when troops are brought into collision with the civil population. It is an extraordinary event, a monstrous event, an event which stands in singular and sinister isolation.

In many past situations not unlike or worse than that faced by Dyer, troops had shown great judgment, he argued, displaying mercy and kindness to those who deserved it and even aiding enemy wounded at the risk of their own lives. They knew how to mete out punishment when called for, but did so with measured restraint. Certainly, in a civil protest, facing comparably less danger than in wartime, they should be even more capable of conducting themselves according to the precepts of British justice. Asquith insisted that "there has never been such an incident in the whole annals of Anglo-Indian history, nor, I believe, in the history of our Empire, from its very inception down to the present day." It was "one of the worst outrages in the whole of our history." Only one supporter of the actions taken against Dyer challenged this interpretation in the Commons debate. Labour MP Ben Spoor rose

> to suggest that Amritsar is not an isolated event any more than General Dyer is an isolated officer. These are not things that can be judged apart, if they resulted from a certain policy that some men have pursued, from a certain mentality that some men seem to possess in India in a most extraordinary degree.[43]

As Spoor insisted, General Dyer's actions in Amritsar and the deep anxieties engendered by the massacre cannot be appreciated in isolation; they must be seen within a much broader national and international context. In the aftermath of the war, revolution seemed to be everywhere and bolsheviks active in every part of the British empire: rebellion in India, in fact, apologists of Dyer maintained, could not be considered apart from revolutionary activity taking place throughout the world, which had as its object the expulsion of Britain from India and from all its other imperial possessions. Movements to throw off British rule in Egypt, Persia, and, closest to home, Ireland, insisted Dyer's defenders and, very often, his opponents, too, must be considered all of a piece. In Amritsar, declared Lord Ampthill, Dyer had faced open rebellion, "rebellion concerted with foreign enemies.... It is all one conspiracy, it is all engineered in the same way, it all has the same object—to destroy our sea power and drive us out of Asia." C. Palmer concurred, insisting that "there is in India, as in other parts of the world, a vast organisation determined to bring down the strength and might of the British Empire." Men like Dyer were ready to fight and die to preserve empire, but should he be punished for his actions, the nation could not expect them to continue to do so. As the Marquess of Salisbury put it, "if your Lordships do not support this Motion you will strike a great blow at the confidence of the whole body of officers throughout your Empire whose business it is to defend the cause of law and order and maintain your Government." "I really wonder how many Members of this House and of His Majesty's Government are really following out the conspiracy to drive the British out of India and out of Egypt?" asked Carson, whose support for Dyer was entirely bound up with his determination to stamp out revolt in Ireland, where the government's efforts to put down the insurgency of the Irish Republican Army were coming to naught, and where police and troops had resorted to unlawful reprisals. The events at Amritsar could not be separated out from the Irish question. "The whole Dyer controversy was a thinly coded discussion of Ireland," notes historian Derek Sayer. Palmer sought the assurance of the Chief Secretary for Ireland, Sir Hamar Greenwood, that General Neville Macready, the officer in charge of the British troops in Ireland, "will be supported by the Government in any action, however fearless, to put down these things and that we will not have a repetition of the Dyer business in Ireland?" The Duke and Duchess of Somerset included with their donation to the Dyer Fund set up by the *Morning Post* their conviction that more men like Dyer would secure the empire against rebellion and sedition. "It is a pity we have not a General Dyer in Ireland at the present time, to crush a conspiracy against British rule," they wrote.[44]

Those who condemned Dyer's actions used precisely this possibility to denounce those who supported him. Lord Birkenhead, for example, asked the Lords to consider how their response would differ if Dyer had fired on white subjects, many of whom, after all, had been involved in protests and demonstrations over the past two years.

Any one who stands here and defends the case of General Dyer should be prepared to defend similar conduct in Glasgow, or Belfast, or Winnipeg. The true view is the only one which is consistent with humanity and the history and greatness of this Empire, and it is that any man who claims membership in, and is a citizen of, this empire, whatever his colour and creed, whatever his geographical location, can look to justice within this Empire.

The Marquess of Crewe drew his colleagues' attention to the "300 or 400 people who were shot at sight because a meeting had been proclaimed. Well, for 'India' read 'Ireland,' " he directed them.

No one will deny, I think that, so far as the maintenance of the law is concerned, the South and West of Ireland are in a considerably worse state than the Punjab ever was; probably in as bad a state as it was ever feared it could be, in April of last year. Yes, for 'Amritsar' read 'Limerick' or 'Ennis,' or some town in the South and West, and conceive a precise repetition of the circumstances there. You may be sure that, after public meetings had been forbidden and a crowd collected to hear a speech, a great many of them would be of the same species as the men who committed the outrages at Amritsar. But who will say that it would be wise, or right, or possible to open fire on a crowd of that kind listening to a speech, and to go on shooting until they were all killed? And yet the parallel seems to me fairly exact; and unless we are to admit...that although it is unfortunate to take life in India in this way, yet the lives of Indian rioters are less important than those of European rioters, you must take the Irish parallel and see what would be said supposing indiscriminate shooting took place in the same way in an Irish town.[45]

For those for whom the Amritsar massacre was a travesty, the actions of General Dyer bode ill for a number of other groups who might excite the armed response of the state. The *Nation* cautioned its readers that "General Dyer is a common type among professional soldiers, and five years of war have weakened all over the world the habitual reluctance of civilized men to kill. There are potential imitators of this man in many a mess-room in India, Egypt, and Ireland." Passing off Dyer's actions as legitimate or necessary, the paper warned, or letting him off with only a slap on the wrist, would embolden those in places like Ireland, who were merely awaiting the moment when they might repeat his example. "What was done in the Punjab, in April, may be repeated in

Dublin to-morrow," it asserted, and then raised the specter of this kind of armed response against Britons at home. "When next a really alarming strike arouses the anger and fears of the circles to which this General belongs," it pointed out, "some fanatic may think it is safe to 'shoot well and strong' at a crowd of English miners."[46] The *Guardian* shared this fear, insisting that "General Dyer's more thorough supporters by no means intend to stop at India... After India, Ireland. After Ireland, British workmen on strike."[47]

They were not far off the mark.

4
Reprisals in Ireland, 1919–1921

> The 'Black and Tans' are after all, every one of them, men who fought in the War.[1]
> We have condemned it at Amritsar. We must condemn it in Ireland.[2]

Amritsar left a profound mark on the national psyche, the events in the Jallianwallah Bagh constituting their own trauma that would reverberate significantly as British politicians took steps to confront the nationalist movement in Ireland. Certainly, as we have seen, Dyer's defenders hoped that the government would not restrain a commander whose ruthlessness was required to bring Irish rebels to heel. But many of those who could not countenance the actions of General Dyer against Indians appeared to find them acceptable when directed against the Irish. What they could not tolerate against Indians many seemed eager to perpetrate against Irish men and women. For the rest, reprisals either could not shake them from the lethargy induced by four years of warfare or they could not be assimilated by a nation suffering from profound collective trauma. Either way, the lawlessness and violence of British forces in Ireland went unchecked for more than a year as a campaign against British subjects regarded, since 1916, as enemies of the British people convulsed the island.

In the spring of 1914, the bill giving home rule to Ireland—passed in 1912 in the teeth of intense Unionist opposition—was due to become law. The northern protestant counties, led by Sir Edward Carson and with the complicity of the Conservative leader, Andrew Bonar Law, refused to accept the legislation and armed themselves in preparation for resistance against the implementation of the act. The Irish Volunteers in the south took steps to meet northern violence with their own, creating a situation that could readily have exploded in catastrophe had not the greater cataclysm of the Great War broken out. The government suspended home rule for the duration of the war, a policy accepted by the parliamentary leader of the Irish party, John Redmond, who sought to present the party in as cooperative a light as possible.

Redmond, however, presided over a party and a set of parliamentary tactics that could no longer claim the allegiance of the Irish people, losing ground to a nationalist movement exemplified by Sinn Féin, for which mere home rule would no longer suffice. On 24 April 1916, members of the Irish Volunteers, an organization seeking to create an Irish republic through revolutionary action, a strategy opposed by Sinn Féin, took to the General Post Office steps in Dublin, declared itself the head of a provisional government, and called for the Irish people to rise up and establish an independent Ireland. Regarded even by its protagonists as a "rhetorical gesture," the Easter Rising, as it came to be called, could boast little support among the population. Its suppression by British forces came swiftly, but not before inexperienced British conscripts, fighting "in New Army-style shoulder-to-shoulder attacks that prefigured the Somme in miniature," "suffered dreadful casualties." The use of field artillery and naval guns on an urban population ensured that civilians would be caught in the crossfire and killed. As one historian has noted, "the psychological reaction of many soldiers (and indeed many civilians) to 'rebels' led to a degree of rough treatment, and in a few cases to something much worse." Army officers resorted to torture and summary executions in some instances.[3]

The rising put down, British authorities took harsh action against the rebels and those they believed to be allied with them. In the excesses of their response—the mass arrests of Sinn Féiners (who had not been involved in either the planning or the carrying out of the rising) and the execution by firing squad of 15 Volunteer leaders—the British mobilized Irish public opinion against their actions and in favor of independence where there had been none to speak of before, leading Irish MP John Dillon to protest in parliament the "river of blood" released upon the innocent people of his country. "The madness of your soldiers," as he put it, in the broader context of repressive measures put in place through martial law, served to provoke demands for self-determination amongst the majority of the Irish population in the south who had taken a neutral position in the past.[4]

In the spring of 1918, faced with an all-out offensive by the Germans on the western front, the British government revisited the question of imposing conscription on Ireland, an issue virtually guaranteed to excite massive opposition. The Irish Volunteers readied themselves to use force to prevent conscription; Sinn Féin took advantage of the threat of conscription to rally a national constituency to its standard. In the general elections held in December 1918, Sinn Féin won 76 seats, as against the six seats held by the Irish Parliamentary party: home rule was rejected by the majority of the Irish electorate in the southern counties in favor of out-and-out independence from Britain. The newly—elected MPs refused to take their seats at Westminster and instead, on 21 January 1919, met in their own assembly, the Dáil Éireann, in Dublin. There they declared themselves the elected representatives of the Irish people and established an Irish republic, pledging to "ourselves and our people to make this declaration effective by every means at our command."[5]

Sinn Féin sought to gain and maintain a peaceable independence from Britain. The Irish Volunteers, by contrast, who saw in the Dáil's Declaration of Independence an imprimatur, began to attack members of the police in Ireland, the Royal Irish Constabulary (RIC), counting them as "armed forces of the enemy." The Dáil had given the Volunteers no such charge, and most Sinn Féiners opposed their actions, but the Volunteers soon fashioned themselves into the Irish Republican Army (IRA), giving rise to the impression that they served as a legitimate force, a "National Army," of the new republic. Throughout 1919 they conducted boycotts against local RIC members, effectively alienating them from the general population; they assaulted the odd policemen unfortunate enough to find himself alone and unprotected; and they raided rural RIC outposts for arms, gradually forcing the RIC from the isolated posts of three to four men they held in the countryside into fewer but larger posts of eight to ten police. Attacks on the larger outposts commenced in January 1920; within six months, the IRA had damaged or destroyed 45 barracks, while more than 400 outposts previously abandoned were burned down as a signal to the population that the British authorities could not control the countryside. Their campaign of violence and intimidation of local populations ensured that the British legal system could no longer function. Sinn Féin courts sprang up to take their place, so that de facto civil administration fell into the hands of the republicans. When the IRA made a failed attempt on the life of Lord French, the Lord Lieutenant of Ireland, on 19 December 1919, the British responded by increasing their military presence in Ireland and trying to chase down the gunmen of the "murder gang," as they called the IRA. For its part, the IRA formed itself into more permanent units—the "flying columns" that organized and carried out larger-scaled ambushes of military and police patrols.[6]

The IRA had succeeded in registering significant RIC losses through the deaths or resignations of its constables, forcing British authorities, who were unable to replenish the ranks through recruitment in Ireland, to seek replacements from among former soldiers in the British population. Right from the start, discipline loomed as a major concern. General Neville Macready, commander of British military forces in Ireland, had wished to recruit a special military force, in which he believed he could more easily instill the necessary discipline. But the government preferred a police force. Macready protested to Churchill,

> even if such a corps could be raised within the time required it would not be satisfactory from the point of view of discipline. Police discipline is too weak in the circumstances now prevailing in Ireland, the more so as the men we may expect to recruit are largely men of the New Army, willing to join up for a short period, who will need the strictest discipline.

He recommended instead "the special enlistment as soldiers of eight garrison battalions. They should be men between the ages of 26 and 35 who have served in the war . . . . all necessary powers as regards discipline will be provided by the Army Act." Macready lost this battle, and a police force under the authority of Major-General Henry Tudor was established in May 1920. It joined with the RIC, but in a move anticipating the confusion and indecision that were to characterize the government's actions throughout, to the profound dismay and frustration of military authorities, the para-military duties of the new force differed from those of the conventional police activities of the RIC. A second "Auxiliary Division" under the command of Brigadier-General Crozier, comprised of ex-officers, joined the new police force in July. Blessed, in this respect, by the dearth of employment among demobilized soldiers, the government's call for police recruits yielded thousands of applicants; some 12,000 signed up between the beginning of January 1920 and the end of August 1922. These men carried out the bulk of the fighting against the IRA; it was they who conducted first unofficial and then official reprisals against the non-combatant population, garnering the hate and fear of the southern Irish that reverberates to this day at the mention of their name, the Black and Tans. The story goes that an insufficient number of uniforms to clothe the new recruits made it necessary to improvise a motley outfit out of military and police uniforms, resulting in a color combination of black and tan. But David Neligan asserts that the dreaded sobriquet derived from "a well-known pack of hounds in Tipperary... known as the Black and Tans (after the colour of the animals)," observing wryly that "it was not to be the last time a police irregular outfit in Ireland bore the name of a hunting pack."[7]

For hunt they did, killing over 200 non-combatants in 1920 alone in what one historian has called "the most ruthless coercion in recent imperial history." Thomas MacCurtain, Lord Mayor of Cork, was shot dead in front of his wife by a group of armed men, later found to be members of the RIC, who had blackened their faces and forced their way into his home. Three other lord mayors were killed the next year in virtually the same circumstances. Between January and June 1921, when a truce between the IRA and British forces came into effect, 17 children, 5 women, and 16 unarmed men were killed in attacks carried out by Black and Tans, 30 of them in April alone.[8] Even if we credit only the cursory reports issued by commanders like Macready, Tudor, or Sir Henry Wilson, the Chief of the Imperial General Staff (CIGS), or statements by politicians like Sir Hamar Greenwood (Chief Secretary of Ireland), Winston Churchill (Secretary of State for War), or David Lloyd George (Prime Minister), all of whom denied in public that reprisals were taking place, the kind and degree of violence meted out to the non-combatant population of Ireland by Black and Tans and members of the armed forces stagger the imagination. Weekly reports from Macready to Greenwood, and from Greenwood to the Situation in Ireland Committee (SIC), comprised of a number of cabinet members and high government officials, testify to regular incidents of arson, beatings, shootings, molestation, rape, murder, and mutilation of the civilian population.[9]

Sir John Anderson, Joint Undersecretary in Dublin Castle, told Thomas Jones, Assistant Secretary to the Cabinet Secretariat, in February 1920 that a publican in Fermoy named Prendergast, a man who had recruited for and fought on behalf of the British during the Great War, had gotten drunk and asserted that money paid to the Discharged Soldiers Society, on which he served, would be put to better use in buying arms for Sinn Féin. "He was taken out of his house," Anderson recounted, "his false teeth were knocked down his throat and then he was thrown over the parapet of a bridge into the Black Water and drowned. Some days afterwards his body was found hanging on a tree." In retaliation for the kidnapping of General Lucas by the IRA, reported Macready on 29 June 1920, "the troops at Fermoy broke out of barracks on Sunday night and did a considerable amount of damage to shops in the Town." "The murder of two Constables in an ambush three miles outside the City of Tuam on the 19th," Greenwood told the SIC was followed by a violent outbreak on the part of the police, who burned and otherwise wrecked a number of houses, shops and other buildings in Tuam, including the Town Hall. The total damage and destruction is estimated at sums varying from £60,000 to £100,000, but no person was injured.

After attacks on constables on 8 September in Tullow,

> the two largest shops in Tullow were set on fire and totally destroyed evidently as an act of retaliation for the outrage. The proprietor of the shops was a loyal Nationalist who was not in any way connected with attacks on the Police and lost a son in the war.

Upon hearing of the murder of Constable Krumm in Galway railway station, "a section of the Police in Galway got out of hand and raided the houses of several prominent Sinn Féiners, one of whom they dragged into the streets and killed." The murder of Constable Burke in Balbriggan

> was immediately followed by a violent outbreak of reprisals by the Police who executed summary vengeance for the death of their comrade by killing two reputed Sinn Féin leaders in Balbriggan and committing extensive destruction of property in that town. Among the buildings which were totally destroyed was the well-known hosiery factory of Messrs. Deedes Templer & Co., which gave employment to a large number of people in the district.

Continued reprisals in October and November resulted in the killing of several civilians, including "a hunchback boy ... shot after Tans failed to find his father in a raid;" "Ellen Quinn of Kiltartan, County Galway, ... killed sitting on her garden wall holding a child in her arms when a policeman took a pot shot from a passing lorry;" "two priests ... [and a] young curate in Galway, Fr Griffin, ... fished out of a bog with a hole in his ear," as Tim Coogan described them. These culminated in "the shocking murder of Canon Magner and another innocent civilian near Dunmanway on the 15th instant," which, Greenwood told the SIC, "was in every way a most deplorable affair."[10]

Men involved in the reprisals gave chilling accounts of their actions. Duncan Duff said of his time in the ranks of the Black and Tans, "a veritable Reign of Terror rode, bloody-footed, through the seemingly-peaceful plains and hills of Erin. Hooded, secret Murder stalked everywhere. Bloody, flaming reprisals were followed by bloodier, grimmer counter-reprisals." He told of an incident in Dublin when the petrol truck he was in was fired on. He returned fire. "My bullet shattered a shop-window behind the man" he had aimed at; "the air was filled with whining, shrieking splinters of steel.... Up and down the street hummed and buzzed the bullets of our angry men firing at a few running figures, but no one appeared to be any the worse for our fusillade." His casual remark belies the terror his actions, repeated day after day, generated amongst Dubliners. After another ambush, "the usual thing happened, the crowds either dived into shops or threw themselves flat on the ground, whilst we fired at everything moving and had the satisfaction of killing a couple of men." After the murder of Detective Inspector Blake, his pregnant wife, and three officers of the 17th Lancers, "shot to pieces, some of them at close range with a sporting-gun, than which no weapon delivers a more ghastly wound," Duff described the "Red Terror [that] stalked the streets of the little western Irish town that night. A terrible tale and one that both sides have reason to hope will soon be forgotten, but, at the time, it was one that made that bitter warfare all the more embittered."[11]

In June 1921, the IRA and the government arrived at a truce, which was supposed to bring the attacks and reprisals to an end. During the truce, however, an uprising broke out in a prison. The RIC reestablished order; prisoners retreated to their cells; and a number of Black and Tans exploded in rage. "It was in the cells that most of the injuries were inflicted by the angry Constabulary," Duff recalled, "with the result that filled stretcher after filled stretcher was taken away." He saw "one unfortunate civilian savagely clubbed by the butt-end of a rifle" by a Black and Tan. Later during the truce, in Galway, a fight broke out at town hall dance, to which the Auxiliaries were refused entry. "Thoroughly infuriated" by the sight of a man who had purportedly "been the cause of the death of several men of the R.I.C.," Black and Tans grabbed him, took him around to the back of the building, and "whilst two men kept electric torches playing on him, the rest 'fell in' as a makeshift firing squad. As they brought their rifles to their shoulders a flying figure burst through the line, and was shown by the wavering beams of the torches to be our Divisional Commissioner." With some difficulty, he was able to prevent the execution from taking place.[12]

Measures such as these sickened some members of the British forces in Ireland. On 16 December 1920, an Auxiliary wrote to his mother about the infamous burning and looting of Cork in which I took a reluctant part. We did it all right never mind how much the well intentioned Hamar Greenwood would excuse us. In all my life I have never experienced such orgies of murder, arson and looting as I have witnessed during the past 16 days with the RIC Auxiliaries. It baffles description.... Many who witnessed similar scenes in France and Flanders say, that nothing they had experienced was comparable to the punishment meted out to Cork.... Reprisals are necessary... but there is a lot which should not be done.

This Auxiliary also spoke of the murder of Canon Magner on 15 December 1920.

On our arrival here from Cork one of our heroes held up a car with a priest and a civilian in it and shot them through the head without cause or provocation.... The brute who did it has been sodden with drink for some time and has been sent to Cork under arrest for examination by experts in lunacy. If certified sane he will be court-martialled and shot. The poor old priest was 65 and everybody's friend.

Greenwood told the House on 3 March 1921 that an inquiry had been conducted and that "these cadets were in no way responsible for the crime, and that no action was called for in their case." An army officer who, Sir Henry Wilson attested, had "greatly distinguished himself in the War," wrote to the CIGS on 28 September 1920 to protest the reprisals undertaken not just by the Black and Tans but by members of the military as well. Describing himself as "out and out for King and Empire," he deplored the practice of

importing crowds of undisciplined men who are just terrorising the country. Shooting unfortunate helpless people, burning homes on a large scale and committing brigandage of the worst description... There are other things going on which—alas—this dear old army is ordered to do, foreign to all our high traditions, and other things... too detestable and revolting to contemplate at which the heart of any man who loves these people as I do, must rebel and revolt.... Do, I implore you, help the likes of me before I am driven out of the Army.[13]

Observers described in harrowing detail the reprisals conceded by military and political officials. A *Times* correspondent told of a reprisal that took place in Trim on 27 September 1920. "Two hundred of the 'Black and Tans' entered the little town of Trim early this morning," he telegraphed to his editor,

> singled out the shops and business establishments of those residents alleged to be in sympathy with Sinn Féin, and ransacked, pillaged, and burned all. At noon to-day when I visited the town it had all the appearance of a bombarded town in the war zone of France. Furniture is piled on the main street, houses are still smouldering, and the people are panic-stricken. Two young men are lying in the local hospital, having been shot by the military. . . . one lad of 16, George Griffin, was shot through the groin, while another lad, named James Kelly, was shot in the leg. . . . A tailor. . . was taken into the street and asked where his Sinn Féin sons were. He replied he did not know. A bayonet it is stated, was placed against his breast and a 'Black and Tan' is alleged to have said, 'Put it through the beggar.' A postman appealed to the men to spare the old man. Then they smashed the door of his house, went through every room and destroyed every article in the place.

Hugh Martin of the *Daily News* reported on an incident at Moher, where

> young Willie Gleeson, when his father was abused for saying truthfully that he had no son named Jim, exclaimed, 'Let them shoot me, father, instead of you.' One of the masked men said: 'This is not the lad.' But another interrupted with, 'He'll do, bring him out.' The young man was then taken out in his shirt, and his dead body was found by the roadside a little later by his mother and sisters.[14]

Lady Augusta Gregory, a nationalist hailing from a prominent protestant family, recorded the 9 November 1920 visit of Malachi Quinn, whose wife, Ellen, had been shot by marauding Black and Tans. He looked

> dreadfully worn and changed and his nerves broken, he could hardly speak when he came in. There had been aeroplanes flying very low over the place all day and as he came from Raheen one had swooped and fired 3 shots over him. He believes they shot her on purpose— they came so close. . . . It is true the messenger sent for a Doctor was shot from another lorry, wounded in the leg.

Of the outbreak by the Highlanders recounted by Macready in a report to Greenwood, Lady Gregory recorded on 24 November 1920,

> Marian went to pay the bills in Gort yesterday. They told her the Highlanders had come there and had 'done bad work the evening before' beating men, driving them before them, following them even into the Chapel... P. today says to me they are a 'bad crowd'—they beat women and children as well as men, with the butts of their rifles.... The postman told Marian this morning that the officers of the Highlanders told the people last night it would be on their own heads if anything happened, as the men 'are let go free to do what they like for their last evening in the town.' So everyone left the street, and shops and houses were all locked.

On 9 October 1920, Lady Gregory's physician, Dr Foley, arrived to take care of her granddaughter's broken arm.

> He said 'there was some bad work last night.... Those Black and Tans that were in Clarenbridge went on to Maree... They dragged three men out of their houses there and shot them—Keene and two others. They are not dead, they were wounded, I was sent for to attend them, then they set fire to some of the houses and burned them down.'... He said 'I used not to believe the stories of English savagery whether written or told, I thought they were made up by factions but now I see that they are true'—he said also 'they are savages, they are out for loot.'[15]

Although the molestation and rape of women—"the most serious charge that can be laid at the door of any white man"—was vociferously denied by Greenwood in the House of Commons, the diaries of Lady Gregory attest that these "outrages" did indeed take place. Her 1 October 1920 entry detailed an account by a neighbor, who

> told me today 'There did two car loads of the Black and Tans come into Gort late yesterday evening—they were a holy fright shouting and firing. They broke into houses and searched them, and they searched the people in the street, women and girls too that were coming out from the chapel, that they came running down the street in dread of their life... at Ardrahan... they kept the boys running up and down the road for near an hour and a half and they all but naked

while they were chasing them up and down, and girls the same way. It is a holy crime—it is worse than Belgium,'

he charged, alluding to the tales of rape and mutilation of Belgian women by invading Germans that had been marshalled to justify Britain's entry into the war. On 31 October 1920, Dr Foley returned to Gregory's home to check on his patient. "He was very excited," she recalled,

> and he said that at Clarenbridge they had got drunk and had assaulted a widow. And a man there,—Casey—had come to him yesterday saying 'Don't let your Misses walk on the road, they are out for drink and women,' and said he and his sons had been dragged from their houses, put against the wall and while held there his two daughters were assaulted. Foley thinks the attempt succeeded to violate them.

On a subsequent visit, Foley told her that "the family of the girls violated by the Black and Tans wish it hushed up. There has been another case of the same sort in Clare—but there also it is to be kept quiet." Men, too, were subjected to sexual molestation. "Lady Fingall tells me of the illtreatment [*sic*] of young men by the military in Mayo," Lady Gregory recounted on 11 July 1921, "told her by Sister Bernard of the Foxford Industries. They were stripped naked on a bridge, beaten with rifles, indecently treated and then thrown over the bridge into the river. They escaped alive but with what memories!"[16]

In December 1920, an act of especially gruesome violence was carried out against two brothers, Patrick and Henry Loughnane. Over a period of a week, as Lady Gregory's diary shows, the fate of the men was the subject of terrible speculation. On 3 December 1920, she recorded, "whispers on the countryside tell of anxiety, Marian tells me, about the two Shanaglish boys who were taken away and have not been heard of. And the men who took them—military or Black and Tans—came back with them to Coen's in Gort, and bought a rope." Three days later, she recorded,

> J., says 'there was news brought to him last night that the bodies of those two Loughnane boys were found, near Murty Sheehan's cross roads, in a pond that is back from it towards Ballindoreen. It is said they had no clothes on them, and had the appearance of being choked. It looks very bad, but those Black and Tans can do what they

like, and no check on them. Look how the Head Constable was afraid to take a deposition from Mrs. Quinn before she died, and he in the house... It is true about the Loughnanes.... The flesh was as if torn off the bones.'

The next day, 7 December 1920, Lady Gregory heard that "the two Loughnane boys could not be recognised"—"that the bodies looked as if they had been dragged after the lorries."

J. says... 'It is not known for certain how they came by their death. There are some say they were burned. For Murphy went out into the pond after they were found to bring them in, and when he took a hold of the hand of one of them it came off in his hand.'

Tim Coogan has viewed the postmortem pictures of the Loughnane brothers. "All I will say," he writes, "is I hope the fire which destroyed the lower parts of their bodies was not started before they died." Mutilations accompanied death in a number of instances: Coogan cited one case in which Black and Tans caught six unarmed IRA men in Cork. They could be "identified by their clothes only when their bodies were handed over to their relatives. One had had his heart cut out, another his skull battered in, a third his nose cut off, a fourth his tongue."[17]

Though they repeatedly denied that reprisals took place, government officials not only knew of them, as we have seen, they excused them, justified them, often approved of them, and may well have instigated them. Wilson wrote in his diary of 12 July 1920 that through what he regarded as a "counter-murder association," the force that would become the Black and Tans, Churchill "evidently had some lingering hope of our rough handling of the Sinn Féins." Six weeks later, Macready confided to Wilson that he believed Churchill was behind the initiation of reprisals. "Strictly between ourselves," he wrote on 1 September 1920, "I am quite sure that Winston has encouraged Tudor in that particular line, from what I heard the former say at a certain Cabinet Meeting." Wilson concurred, responding to Macready on 2 September 1920, "yes, I am quite sure from the very disconcerted face which Winston assumed when I attacked him about Tudor's people, that Winston himself is probably at the bottom of the mischief and more than likely the originator of the idea." In a "Very Secret Memo from Lt. Col. D.K. Bernard to Macready" about Tralee, Bernard complained that "it is idle to pretend that all the R.I.C. there are under the control of their officers; some of them are either working entirely on their own or are being told unofficially to do things which are then officially ignored." Officials in Dublin Castle, it appears, encouraged the police to carry out reprisals, apparently at the urging of Lloyd George. Sir John Anderson told Thomas Jones in February 1921 that he believed

> that the P.M. was the person really responsible for the policy of reprisals. Anderson had the feeling that whenever Tudor came over to see the P.M. he returned very much strengthened in his policy— that even if not in words yet by atmosphere and suggestion the P.M. conveyed his encouragement to Tudor.

Duncan Duff told of the efforts of the *Weekly Summary*, the paper put out by the Dublin Castle Press Bureau to the RIC, "to rouse our blood," which, he asserted, would have been "laughable had they not been so dangerous." A poem in the 4 March 1921 issue of the paper can only be seen as an urging to violence by lynching. Entitled "Up the Rebels," it read, "They say 'Up the Rebels,'/And high up they soon will be./Higher than they'd hoped for—/A rope swinging from a tree./And the Irish people—/For whom they've filled a bitter cup,/Of misery and loathing—/Will be glad to see them 'Up.' "[18]

From the start, officials in Ireland and members of the government like Churchill, Lloyd George, and Greenwood regarded the reprisals inflicted on the civilian population by British forces as one of the only effective ways to deal with assaults carried out by the IRA. Mark Sturgis, a high-ranking English civil servant in Dublin Castle, recorded in his diary in August 1920 that "we are being urged quietly and persistently that Reprisals are the only thing to put down the Gun men and hearten the police." "There is no doubt we have benefited by them to some extent," he added in October. Wilson recorded in his diary of 22 September 1920 that Black and Tans in three towns "marked down certain Sinn Féiners as actual murderers or instigators & then coolly went & shot them without question or trial. Winston saw very little harm in this." A few days later, Lloyd George declared to three of his cabinet colleagues that the murder of policemen "can only be met by reprisals." Tudor reported that "L.G. is all against burning but not gunning, and told him as much himself." Lloyd George made a more public admission when he told a Guildhall audience on 9 November 1920 that "there is no doubt that at last their patience has given way and there has been some severe hitting back" by the RIC. Because of their actions, he declared, "we have murder by the throat . . . . we had to reorganise the police. When the Government was ready we struck the terrorists and now the terrorists are complaining of terror."[19]

Virtually every military or governmental official and the editorial writers of a number of the mainstream newspapers believed that acts of retaliation by members of the British forces could only be expected, given the conditions under which they had to operate. As Churchill put it,

> the troops and the police bore the strain of the assassinations, for which of course hardly anyone was brought to justice, with exemplary patience for a long time. But at length their distress and indignation led them to take the law into their own hands... it will always be very difficult to persuade armed bodies of men to endure with impassive good humour for any long period being hunted down and murdered one by one.... The unauthorised reprisals grew with the increasing provocation.

He informed the cabinet in November 1920 that he deprecated the "many foolish and wrong things" that had taken place by men "goaded in the most brutal manner" by IRA assaults on them and their comrades. But "finding no redress" for these crimes, he explained, "they take action on their own account." He, for one, could not find it in him to blame them. "Is it to be wondered at," asked Lt-General Hugh Jeudwine, commander of the Fifth Division in Ireland,

> that men, who were not under military discipline and who were driven half mad by seeing their comrades shot down in cold blood, sometimes took the law into their own hands and indulged in unlawful reprisals. It is to be remembered also that these acts of reprisals—they were not numerous—were nearly always directed against individuals who, it was morally certain, had either taken part in, or were in entire sympathy with, the outrage committed.[20]

Being in sympathy with the IRA could get one killed.

The *Weekly Summary* reprinted a constant stream of stories from mainstream papers in which editors or politicians excused—and, arguably, incited further—reprisals as understandable responses by long-suffering policemen to the murder of their comrades. The 8 October 1920 edition reproduced a *Sunday Times* article describing the "admirable discipline and restraint" displayed by the RIC until July 1920, when, after the murder of two policemen, "a large body of police gave way to an uncontrolled impulse of emotion, wrecking a considerable part of" Tuam in County Galway. This "wild outburst of human passion . . . could not have been prevented by any conceivable precautions taken by the Government," the *Times* declared, and "once the tension of self-restraint, which had been for many months strained almost to the breaking point by the provocation received, had snapped, it was inevitable that similar incidents in like circumstances should occur before authority and discipline could be imposed." On 4 March 1921, the *Weekly Summary* carried a *Daily Telegraph* article recounting Greenwood's protestations to the House of Commons that "isolated cases—of murder, it may be," should be placed in the context of the "gallantry of the men who are standing between this House and chaos in Ireland." The Auxiliaries of the RIC, he asserted, were brave, honourable men who were sacrificing their lives to restore peace in Ireland. The 24 June 1921 issue quoted Lloyd George chastising the clergy for speaking out against reprisals.

> It is very easy for men in the tranquillity—and may I also say the security—of the sanctuary to criticise men who are going in hourly peril of their lives and who while walking along the streets or roads, may at any moment witness the stones on their path becoming the blazing messenger of death.[21]

Even General Macready, who disapproved of the methods of the RIC and feared that indiscipline might spread to his troops, allowed that reprisals on the part of men who had lost comrades or commanders were in the proper nature of things. He told Sturgis that

> a regiment that did not try to break out when a story—however untrue—was told them e.g. that one of their comrades had been chucked into the Liffey and shot at in the water, was not worth a damn, and he had to be careful not to make them sullen and take the heart out of them.

He added that "if a policeman put on a mackintosh and a false beard and 'reprised' on his own hook he was damn glad of it." "Under the present conditions," he wrote to Wilson on 1 September 1920, "I am not prepared to take the usual disciplinary action against troops who indulge in retaliation carried out by them in consequence of the murdering of their officers and comrades." But however much he understood the impulses toward retaliation exhibited by men whose comrades or officers were attacked, he baulked at "some of the wild acts of retaliation" that men under the command of "young R.I.C. officers who stick at nothing" were carrying out. He became alarmed by the frequency, senselessness, and degree of violence with which they took place, but in circumstances where the government refused to institute martial law and in which the IRA appeared to have a free hand without fear of official retribution, he hesitated to punish men for fear that even greater acts of indiscipline would result.[22]

Macready despaired of the situation. He wrote to Wilson on 28 August 1920, allowing as how "the action of these 'Black and Tans' of Tudor's makes me every day increasingly anxious. The time will, I feel quite sure, come when the Military will have to interfere." A month later, he repeated his warning. "These 'Black and Tans' are really going too far," he told Wilson.

> If they would confine themselves to killing well known leaders of the Murder Gang when their own officers and comrades are murdered I should remain silent, but this wholesale burning not only does no good, or at least very little, but I am afraid they will get so far out of hand that the day may come when it will require half the British army to get rid of them.

He feared that when that time came, his soldiers might refuse orders "against men who were their own comrades in the War. If the delinquents were old R.I.C. I do not think the Army would have any feelings in the matter, but the 'Black and Tans' are after all, every one of them, men who fought in the War." Although he and Wilson worked hard to impress upon anyone who would listen that it was the police and not the army who carried out reprisals, he knew it could only be a matter of time before the indiscipline spread to his troops. "I see there are more casualties among the Camerons to-day, and I fancy one of these days the Highland blood will get the better of discipline and there will be considerable trouble for S.F.'s whether they be of the peaceful description or the reverse," he admitted to Wilson on 1 September 1920. Then, in a handwritten postscript, he added, "Have just heard the Camerons have wrecked Rucastown [?] . . . If we punish the men for revenging the murder of their officers we shall have mutiny—& quite right too." He wrote to Wilson on 25 September 1920, "You will have seen that they shot at Strickland and missed him . . . . If they had killed him, by this time Cork would probably have been even as Sodom and Gomorrah, and I for one would not have blamed the troops." In the same letter he confessed that the discipline of his troops could not be counted on for too much longer.

> We are sitting on a powder barrel that may go off at any moment. I hope Strickland's action in having these six men arrested will prevent any retaliation on the part of the troops, but I am momentarily expecting to hear that Cork is not quite what it was yesterday.

Three days later, he reiterated his fear that

> if a murder is committed on some fairly senior, popular man like Tudor or Boyd, unless it is know [sic] that the Government are prepared to take effective measures, no power on earth would restrain the troops (I am not concerned with the Police) from breaking out and having something in the shape of a Massacre.[23]

Macready proposed to institute authorized reprisals as a means of bringing the troops and police under control. He informed Wilson on 22 September 1920 that he had "told [General] Strickland and others that they have my permission to let it be known that they will take place under certain conditions, but in the case of the Army it will, of course, be done regularly and 'by numbers.' " One such authorised reprisal occurred

> down at Ennistymon [where] the Royal Scots carried out certain retaliations 'by numbers' under order of the C.O. The men were maddened by the sight of the bodies of the Police who were killed and mutiliated by expanding bullets, and if the C.O. had not done what he did, he would probably not have held his men. The only responsible person was the C.O. And as the Regiment is a good one, and both Brigade and Divisional Commanders consider it was the only course to take, I shall merely tell him not to do it again.

Churchill was convinced that the new policy of authorized reprisals would fail to bring the IRA to its knees; indeed, he recorded in his account of the immediate postwar years that "it speedily proved far less effective than the rough and ready measures of the special police." The policy also raised concerns among some officers of their being prosecuted for taking matters into their own hands, as when Macready reported to Wilson on 14 October 1920 that one of his commanders "may have an idea that he may become a second Dyer." Macready stood by the policy of official reprisals as a necessity if unauthorized reprisals were to be reined in and was prepared to take all responsibility if things were to go afoul. "I have tried to get it into all these people's heads that there will only be one 'Dyer' in this country, and that is myself," he declared.[24]

In this instance, however, some of the politicians like Churchill who had remonstrated so vociferously against General Dyer's actions in India were more than prepared to countenance official attacks that involved machine-gunning and bombing Irish citizens from the air. Wilson wrote to Macready on 13 October 1920 that Churchill "is beginning to agree that the Government must shoulder the responsibility for carrying out reprisals.... the logic of events will force the Government to take over the responsibility of reprisals," at which point, he assumed, "it will be infinitely easier for you to restrain the troops from taking reprisals on their own and comparatively easy for you to jump on any officers or men who carry out reprisals of their own." His confidence was misplaced, for although the government approved a policy of authorized reprisals to go into effect on 1 January 1921, reports of retaliation by Black and Tans and Auxiliaries continued to pour in, finally compelling Lloyd George, for political reasons, to upbraid Greenwood. "I am not at all satisfied with the state of discipline of the Royal Irish Constabulary and its auxiliary force," he wrote to his Chief Secretary on 25 February 1921.

> Accounts reach me from too many and too authoritative quarters to leave any doubt in my mind that the charges of drunkenness, looting, and other acts of indiscipline are in too many cases substantially true.... I need not tell you that the accumulating evidence that in certain sections of the Irish police there are men who are no longer the guardians of the law, but are themselves guilty of unlawful acts against the population it is their duty to protect, is causing grave uneasiness in the public mind.... As you know, I have given to yourself and to your subordinates my full and unswerving support. But it is vital that the violence and indiscipline which undoubtedly characterise certain units in the R.I.C. should be terminated in the most prompt and drastic manner.[25]

Reluctantly, the government turned to the extension of martial law as perhaps the only way to both act against the IRA and keep reprisals by the Black and Tans and Auxiliaries in check. The government had imposed it in the south-west of Ireland in November 1920, but only after long soul-searching; with the example of Dyer so fresh in their minds, few politicians wished to take the step. As Balfour noted in a cabinet meeting in July 1920, "This is going to be attacked in the country and the Dyer debate has not helped us to govern by soldiers." Macready had strongly opposed it initially, fearing that without the support of the British public, which he believed would not be forthcoming, martial law could not work, but the alarm he felt at the behavior of the Crown forces compelled him to change his position. Conditions being what they were, the danger of army and police breaking out was too great, he feared. "As you know," he wrote to Wilson on 25 September 1920,

> I have fought all along against Martial Law because I had doubts whether the country on your side of the water would stand it, but I see now that unless some step in that direction is taken, ... a far worse state of affairs might arise if prominent officials are done in. For instance, take Tudor. I believe if they killed Tudor that there would hardly be a village within ten miles of a 'Black and Tan' detachment that would not be in flames within twenty-four hours.

He followed the next day with a stronger entreaty. "We must have Martial Law in order to protect us against Police," he urged Wilson. "It may sound strange but it is so . . . . we cannot go on like this . . . The Police I hear killed about 30 for the murder of the 5 police and the R.M. at Ennistymon."[26]

But the government hesitated, willing to place the area around Dublin under martial law but not prepared to apply it to the entire country, for fear of alienating the British public, especially in the context of the Amritsar massacre. Finally, events on the ground forced the government to acquiesce in the demands of the military. As Wilson explained to his former aide General Rawlinson on 18 May 1921,

> in Ireland we have had one of the worst week-ends since the beginning of the rebellion, and it is perfectly clear to me that unless the 'Frocks' shout out at the top of their voices and get England on their side, and then really set to work to stamp out this vermin we shall lose Ireland, and with the loss of Ireland we have lost the Empire. I want permission from the 'Frocks,' the moment England gets temporarily quiet again, to send over between 20 and 30 battalions, from here, some more cavalry, guns, aeroplanes, wireless, tanks, armoured cars etc. to place the whole of Ireland under Martial Law, and hand it all over to Macready.[27]

The Irish Situation Committee met within the week and produced a draft of its conclusions at its 26 May 1921 session. Amazingly, the rationale for extending martial law was to gain control not over the Irish rebels but over the police and armed forces. "The placing of the Police under Martial Law would lead to a strengthening of discipline in that Body," the committee declared.

> The extension of Martial Law will obviate the necessity for authorised reprisals, which are at present resorted to as a safety valve for the feeling amongst the soldiers and police. If the Crown Forces feel that rebels who are caught carrying arms will be subject to the severest penalties they will be far less likely to get out of hand. Reprisals are particularly objectionable now because they had lead [*sic*] to counter reprisals by Sinn Féin.

Macready told the committee that

> he felt that he was losing the confidence of his men and he asked the Committee and the Government to bear in mind the personal feeling of the tools which the Government were using. If they did not do so, those tools would break in their hands. It must be 'all out' or some quite different policy.

The proposed terms of martial law were draconian: any Sinn Féiner in the 26 counties of the south found with firearms would be subject to execution after a "drumhead court martial," a procedure supported by Greenwood on the grounds that "the quicker men were executed the more palatable executions were to the Irish and the less trouble they cause in this country." "Any man found with revolvers or bombs would be shot at once." "Persons found actively engaged in hostilities with arms or explosives will be executed on the spot after trial by drumhead Court Martial.... the extreme penalty will be exacted to the utmost." Arthur Balfour agreed with "the substance of the announcement" of martial law, but feared that the way it was to be presented was "unnecessarily terrifying. The announcement painted the Government's policy in a sanguine hue," he protested. Macready replied that he had presented the terms in such a way purposefully, "principally to harden the troops and the Policy and to prepare the people in this country and in Ireland for what would happen." Macready warned that "if Martial Law were fully enforced on and after July 14th, there might be as many as one hundred men shot in a week."[28]

Lloyd George's government apparently realized that such a state of affairs would not be tolerated by the country, and within three weeks made what Churchill regarded as one of the most sudden and total reversals of policy in modern British history. Unable to stomach any longer methods that Lord Addison called "repugnant" and H.A.L. Fisher described as "evil" and "degrading," the government initiated truce talks with the IRA.

Virtually all the Black and Tans and Auxiliaries who were responsible for the bulk of the violence against the Irish had served in the British Army, many of them, undoubtedly, having seen action, where, Churchill reminds us, they "had been through a mill of prolonged inconceivable pressures and innumerable tearing teeth. To all, sudden and violent death, the woeful spectacle of shattered men and dwellings was, either to see in others or expect and face for oneself, the commonest incident of daily life." Upon the end of hostilities, observed journalist Phillip Gibbs, soldiers who had just a short time before been defending their country against the German enemy turned on their officers in a "revolt against all discipline."

> Soldiers... ran amok in camps and towns, attacked police, looted shops, stormed town halls, fought in a brutal, demoniacal way with the guardians of law and order. There was something unreasonable in these sudden gusts of fury, something that looked like madness, as in the case of young officers even who took part in these affrays and afterwards swore, as I think sincerely, that they could remember nothing of how they came to be mixed up in the rioting or what they had done. It was just a sudden lack of self-control, a sudden uprising of ungovernable and unreasoning passion.

Gibbs blamed their behavior on the "disease which doctors called 'shell-shock,' though it afflicted men and women far behind the lines, aloof from shell-fire, the long nagging of the war upon the nervous system, until it was all worn and frayed, the high tension of war excitement which suddenly snapped when the Armistice was signed." "In several cases considerable bodies of men were for some days entirely out of control," Churchill recalled, a situation repeated, according to Gibbs,

> during the great coal strike in England [when] the government called up the Reservists to maintain order in case of rioting by the miners and the army of unemployed. For the most part the miners

behaved like lambs, but at Aldershot, Woolwich, and other places, the Reservists, all 'veterans' of the Great War, broke bounds, and started looting and rioting until they were dispersed by cavalry.[29]

The violence carried out by the Black and Tans in Ireland can be attributed in part to the traumas they experienced during wartime, exacerbated by the unprecedented nature of guerrilla warfare in Ireland that heightened the sense of the unknowability of the situation. Certainly contemporaries believed that the war played a big part, seeing in many of the outbreaks of violence "the inevitable effect of the four years of war on the men of both forces." Brigadier-General C.B. Thomson, who served as military advisor to the Labour Commission investigating events in Ireland, believed that the violence was carried out by "victims of the war... suffering from nerve strain." We have tantalizingly hints from Black and Tans themselves that their actions were a product of the war experiences they had undergone. Lady Gregory, for instance, heard from a friend in Galway that even though a Black and Tan to whom her nurse was engaged "had had shell shock," he insisted that "I am not like the others—I am a university man and it was a great shock to me to find what sort of men they are. I am not like them, I don't like killing people." In his memoirs Duncan Duff recounted harrowing experiences from the war years, using much of the same language mobilized by the veterans we saw in Chapter 1. He began his naval service in 1916, at the age of 14, aboard the transport ship *Thracia*, where he experienced many terrifying incidents that imprinted themselves on his psyche. When he was 15, the *Thracia* was struck by a torpedo. "Out on the deck there was an indescribable scene," he recalled.

My bare foot slithered in something warm and sticky, the blown—asunder body of a sailor who had received the full blast of the explosion.... There was a sudden, all-pervading roar of waters [sic] and the ship slithered away from under my feet. It was not more than ninety seconds from the time of the explosion, and I felt myself swept helplessly away by the rushing water.

Picked up days later and delivered to a French destroyer, he "was called on deck to identify the bodies of several of my shipmates."[30]

After a stay in Ireland "to recover from the terrific experiences through which I had just passed," he returned to duty. On one voyage, as his ship tried to escape from a submarine, "I had both bones of my right leg shattered." In 1918, at age 16, Duff was on board the transport ship *Flavia* along with American nurses, Serbian soldiers, and "several hundred horses" when it was hit by a torpedo. "The Serbians, or a great part of them, had gone mad with panic, and the horses were swelling the terror-stricken din. By the time I gained the deck, ... I found a fierce fight in progress between the seamen and the terror-mad soldiers." As the ship began to sink, "the squealing of hundreds of horses that knew their death was upon them and the shouts of the Serbians rendered the morning hideous." Crew and passengers took to the lifeboats, and

almost immediately the bubbling, frothy, milky vortex was dotted with hundreds of swimming horses, who, seeing the boats, made directly for them. The heavily-laden craft could not be pulled away in time, and rapidly the swimming animals gained on us.... Wildly the boats rolled as we fought off the maddened horses with oars, boat-hooks and axes.

On board the *Caronia,* part of a fleet transporting Americans to Brest from New York, the convoy was struck by the flu. "There were hundreds of sick, gasping, coughing, spitting, dying." Duff recalled. "The floors were covered with sputum and vomit so thickly, that, as the vessel rolled, it washed up, inches deep, against the bulkheads." In the five and a half days it took to cross the Atlantic, 78 men died.[31]

Duff described his experiences of the war as "a bad chapter, despair, disease, vice and death, best forgotten," but, as was the case for so many Great War veterans, the effort to expel the memories and visions from consciousness would fail. "My nerves called aloud for a rest and an easement from horror," he admitted. "After all, I had seen and suffered things between the ages of fifteen and eighteen, that few boys are called upon to face." He entered a monastery, where the regimen was "peaceful, well ordered and regulated. Undoubtedly it was the finest thing that could have happened to me to soothe my war-jangled nerves." Tiring of the life of contemplation, however, he joined the new RIC force, and soon found himself in a place where peace, order, and regulation were supplanted by violence, chaos, and confusion, a situation virtually calculated to drive war-weary, shell-shocked men over the edge. Contemporaries constantly remarked that Black and Tans seemed to commit their atrocities while drunk, a classic behavior of trauma victims seeking to numb their feelings of fear and helplessness.[32]

The wartime traumas of men like Duff were exacerbated by the sheer unknowability and unpredictability characteristic of guerilla warfare in Ireland. Guerilla warfare made it impossible for the British to distinguish combatant from non-combatant, a situation in which clear, definitive differences between and among groups could not be observed. Men complained that "the rebels," who wore no uniforms and could easily masquerade as a "harmless worker in the field, loafer at street corners, or assistant in a shop," might, without a moment's notice, become transformed into gunmen intent upon ending their lives.

> A group of men playing the Irish national game of pitch and toss by the roadside is so common a sight that it was a simple matter for a party of rebels intent on attacking a small patrol to camouflage themselves in this way. Men apparently engaged at work on the land could without difficulty form themselves into an ambush along the hedges on the approach of troops being signalled by a scout.

Women and children compounded the confusion by aiding the nationalist cause. Officially exempt from search by soldiers and police—a nice bit of chivalry often honored only in the breach, as we have seen—they might be the conduits for arms, ammunition, or information. "The smile of an Irish girl may be the lure to a death of agony," wrote an officer in the Black and Tans in the *Weekly Summary*. "The very street boys are bred to murder and organised as spy scouts." Confounded by the possibility, for example, of a "Woman with Lewis Gun" in Blarney, as the 21 January 1921, issue of the *Weekly Summary* trumpeted in a headline, Crown forces operated in a state in which all the signs that would have oriented them had been obliterated.[33]

Faced with this kind of warfare, where "all the Crown Forces are in the 'front line' all the time;" where "there was . . . no defined theatre of war, since non-combatants and loyal persons were intermingled with rebels in every district; there was no 'front line' or 'No Man's Land';" where, because police and soldiers could not know who was friend and who was foe, "all civilians had to be regarded as potential enemies." That indistinguishable mass we saw so often in accounts of Amritsar had its counterpart in the conviction that "every Irishman was a Sinn Féiner," that "the bulk of the people were our enemies." Added to that was the belief that the Irish had not only shirked their duty in the Great War but had, in fact, explicitly harmed the British war effort. The conviction among many participants in or apologists for the reprisals that the Irish had let the British down by resisting conscription in 1918 or, more dramatically, through the Easter Rising of 1916 served to justify the murderous attacks on the Irish Catholic population. As the *Weekly Summary* of 3 June 1921 quoted Greenwood as stating, we cannot forget the bitter periods during the war, when the Irish rebellion made us keep 100,000 troops in Ireland, and which made us sacrifice the lives of brave boys of this country because of the hostility of those Sinn Féiners. That lesson has not been forgotten by the British Government.

Macready, for example, confessed to loathing the Irish "with a depth deeper than the sea and more violent than that which I feel against the Boche." And although Henry Wilson protested that the violence against Britain was the product not of the people of Ireland as a whole, but of a small band of insurgents, he regarded the nationalists as "as much an enemy to England as were the Boche." Journalist Hugh Martin noted that the Black and Tans "believe that the Irish 'let the British down,' and they are not averse from getting their own back in their own way."[34] Seeing in the Irish, consciously or not, people who may have contributed to their wartime traumas could not have helped British soldiers and police keep an even keel.

The precariousness of the psyche in such a situation could readily produce behavior designed to stave off the real threat of annihilation. "Maddened by the sight of their murdered comrades and the constant danger to their own lives," as the 15 April 1921 issue of the *Weekly Summary* put it, police and soldiers engaged in violence against non-combatants that should be regarded not as reprisals, the paper insisted, but as "outbursts." The murder of Canon Magner may well have been one such outburst by a man whose fragile hold on himself was attenuated to a tragic degree as a result of his experiences in Ireland. He "is said to be one of the party recently bombed and to be mad," wrote Sturgis, adding that if he was mad, "surely those responsible for leaving him loose on the world in charge of a party armed to the teeth should take his place in the dock."[35]

The daily uncertainty faced by forces confronted by an unknowable, unpredictable threat was made worse by the failure of the government to articulate a clear, purposeful plan of action. Lloyd George sought to follow a course that combined coercion with conciliation, a strategy that he hoped would alienate the IRA from the rest of the population and enable him to defeat the armed insurgency while still maintaining Ireland for the empire. "Three weapons were used simultaneously by the Government," Duff pointed out,

namely severe and ruthless coercion, martial law, and secret negotiations with and concessions to the Sinn Féin leaders. Any of them might have had good results, if followed whole-heartedly, but their combination resulted in mystifying and misleading every single party in Ireland. Coercive measures were almost invariably taken too late, and were sometimes weakened after their imposition. It has been said frequently that an Irishman only understands firmness, by which severity is usually meant. What an Irishman, like almost everyone else, does understand, is consistency and he respects, though he may not always like, moral courage. No one, not even an Irishman, appreciates a 'slap and stroke' policy.

An amorphous, seemingly incoherent policy compounded the incoherence felt by individuals. As Duff put it, they were "egged on to be brutal and tyrannizing one day, imprisoned and dismissed the service the next if we dared to speak roughly to our enemies."[36]

At the level of military operations, the conduct of this policy produced disorganization, miscommunication, and confused lines of authority. Walter Long, chair of the Irish Situation Committee, protested the lack of

clear definition being given to the various officers holding the most important administrative posts in the Irish Government as to the extent of their authority. The precise duties of the military and police are obscure and in some cases the police are considered to be under the military and in others the military under the police. The Committee are strongly of the opinion that the duties and responsibilities of the officers who administer these two bodies should be so defined as to admit of no confusion.

Commanders complained bitterly about the vacillation of policy, "the lack of an objective," "the present divided control by military and police, which is enforced by different authorities in different ways, according to very diverse standards, and often with more than questionable justice or even advantage." They yearned for "sound and well understood policy—the clear expression of a firm determination to bring about a certain defined state of affairs," for "clear and definite orders," for "co-ordinated effort, unity of command." Their pleas read like the descriptions offered by Herbert Read, Ford Maddox Ford, and Richard Aldington—without coherence, without a plan, there could be no narrative structure to help them make sense of what was happening.[37]

At home, the acts of reprisals against non-combatant Irish seemed to have elicited little response from the British public for almost a year. The newspapers reflected the broad range of political opinion in expected ways—the *Daily News*, Manchester *Guardian* and *Westminster Gazette*, as befit their Liberal leanings, deprecated the violence in Ireland; *The Times*, representing moderate Conservative opinion, gave tentative support to government actions, while the *Morning Post*, the *National Review*, and the *Spectator* cheered them on more vociferously. The *Daily Herald*, speaking for Labour, could countenance no force whatsoever. But the public itself remained aloof. H.H. Asquith pronounced himself "amazed and ashamed of the lethargy and the indifference with which the English people regarded these things." Gibbs lamented

the indifference of the mass of English people to the reign of terror in Ireland. It was not that they hated Sinn Féiners, or upheld the policy of reprisals by the Black and Tans. Theoretically the ranks of Labour were sympathetic to the Irish rebels, and hostile to the Government's policy of coercion. Actually they did not care. The dreadful episodes of that struggle, ambushes and arson, assassinations by this side and the other, men dragged out of their beds and shot before their wives and children, the hanging of boys in batches, all that horror of guerilla warfare and military repression, left English psychology stone cold or just mildly interested.[38]

This lack of reaction on the part of the British was unprecedented, Gibbs claimed, a product of the agonizing war years just concluded. "Before the war," he insisted,

a storm of passion would have swept over England. There would have been a fierce partisanship, wild meetings, passionate protests, mob demonstrations. After the war only small groups of 'intellectuals' excited themselves about the state of Ireland. In the streets I used to read newspaper placards with a sense of sickness: 'Cork in Flames'—'British Soldiers ambushed near Dublin'—'Five more Policemen shot in Ireland'—'Extensive Raids in Irish Towns'—'More Creameries destroyed by Crown Forces.' But the crowds went by, indifferent, in the Strand. No flame of indignation lit up their lacklustre eyes.... The killing of women in Ireland by British soldiers 'shooting up' Irish villages did not raise a flicker of interest among the general public in England, nor command more than a few paragraphs in English papers.[39]

One manifestation of collective trauma is, simply, refusal to face a situation that conjures up the original injury. Given the coverage of and energy expended on the Amritsar massacre, I think we have to see the indifference to Black and Tan atrocities in Ireland as the response of a country that could not face one more blow.

Ultimately, however, roused by increasing coverage in the press, especially by accounts of the sack of Balbriggan by British forces in September 1920, the public began to take notice, and it did not like what it saw. This time opinion did not break along predictable political lines—instead, the conservative and liberal press alike decried the reprisals that seemed to be occurring every day. Liberal and Labour politicians denounced the reprisals and the government policies that appeared to excuse them; some Conservatives joined them in their opposition, convinced that such behavior could not serve British interests. The actions of the Black and Tans and the official reprisals of the army provoked the same kind of debate about Britishness raised by Amritsar. Not surprisingly, echoes of that debate reverberate in this one: outrage that England, "the champion of small peoples, the friend of liberty, pledged to the self-determination of peoples, should adopt a Prussian policy in Ireland after a war in which, after all, hundreds of thousands of Irishmen had fought for the Empire." The Labour Commission and others protested against these acts of violence against subjects of the empire. "Ireland is still part of the United Kingdom, not territory occupied in war," protested J. Annan Bryce to *The Times*. It is, insisted a number of intellectuals—Arnold Bennett, W. Lyon Blease, Wilfrid Seawen Blunt, Edward Carpenter, G.K. Chesterton, Margaret Llewelyn Davies, Walter de la Mare, G. Lowes Dickinson, Havelock Ellis, E.M. Forster, Roger Fry, Jane Harrison, Ford Maddox Huefner [Ford], Augustus John, J.M. Keynes, Rose Macaulay, H.J. Massingham, Alice Meynell, Harold Munro, Gilbert Murray, Charles S. Myers (Director of the Psychological Laboratory), Sir Arthur Quiller-Couch, Lady Rhondda, Dorothy Richardson, Siegfried Sassoon, May Sinclair, J. Arthur Thomson, Sybil Thorndike, A.J. Toynbee, and Virginia Woolf, among others—who put their name to a protest against British behavior in Ireland, "a nation that co-equally with ourselves has inherited our traditions of individual liberty." The Labour Commission concluded,

> Things are being done in the name of Britain which must make her name stink in the nostrils of the whole world. The honour of our people has been gravely compromised. Not only is there a reign of terror in Ireland which should bring a blush of shame to every British

citizen, but a nation is being held in subjection by an Empire which has proudly boasted that it is a friend of small nations.[40]

"We are not a brutal people," protested Gibbs. "We are, taking us all in all, a good-hearted, tolerant, and generous people," He attributed the very un-English actions of the government and the armed forces to one particular kind of Englishman,

> the old type of John Bull Englishman, hardly exaggerated by his cari-cature, but utterly unrepresentative of the nation as a whole—hard in his Imperialism, narrow in his Protestantism, reactionary against any effort of change or progress, sure that the Englishman of his own type is the noblest effort of God, disliking all aliens, including Irish, Welsh, and Scotch, and a firm believer in 'resolute rule,' with machine-guns and tanks for all rebellious people, such as native races, and working-men who want more wages. He was the defender of the Amritsar massacre.

Possessed of great power and holding the levers of political life, "that type of man is still to be found in many places and classes of English life, and it was his type which supported Sir Hamar Greenwood and the Prime Minister's Tory masters in their policy." He was representa-tive of many on the Irish Situation Committee, who believed that the Irish outside the seven northern counties were inclined to support, or lacked the moral courage to prevent, "a campaign of outrage and mur-der." Military officials, noted the author of the 5th Division history, went further, asserting that 90 percent of the Irish people were "mur-derers or sympathised with murder." "Judged by English standards the Irish are a difficult and unsatisfactory people," it declared.

> Their civilisation is different and in many ways lower than that of the English. They are entirely lacking in the Englishman's distinctive respect for the truth and their answers are usually coloured by a desire to say what their questioner wishes.... Many were of a degenerate type and their methods of waging war were in most cases barbarous, influenced by hatred and devoid of courage.

Wilson thought them "vermin," Macready a "cancer," while Churchill professed relief that the Irish would no longer be a part of British par-liamentary life. Had Sinn Féin taken the seats they won in the 1918 election, he declared, "for a long time in our Parliamentary life and Party electioneering, there would be gnawing at the very vitals of the Empire, an untamed, untutored band of haters, carrying into English public life a malignity unknown for generations—even for centuries."[41]

But finally, even the John Bull Englishman described by Gibbs could not be squared with the kinds of actions taken by the British in Ireland and had to be displaced onto those who were not really English. Gibbs ascribed the behavior of the British in Ireland, who engaged in "action and policy contrary... to our traditions of honour and justice," to the Chief Secretary, Sir Hamar Greenwood, "a Canadian Jew, who, in my judgment, has done more to dishonour the British Empire than any living man."[42]

As had been true of Amritsar, the events in Ireland were intricately bound up with other issues and concerns, and policies and practices there seemed, for many, to have profound implications for other areas of British imperial and domestic affairs. Over and over again, for instance, Wilson despaired that he could not provide Macready with sufficient troops to get the job done. Partly that was a consequence of the need to keep troops in Europe to maintain the armistice; partly it was owing to the dispersal of troops to parts of the world like Mesopotamia and Palestine that Britain now claimed an interest in. Perhaps most importantly, however, was the conviction on the part of politicians and military men that armed force would have to be mobilized against striking workers at home. The industrial situation, especially that in the coal mines, posed a major problem for the government, reducing it to handling the troop shortage in Ireland as best it could. The intimation of the Irish Situation Committee that the extension of martial law was contingent upon amassing sufficient armed force was only one such expression of concern: "The Committee agreed:—That reinforcements should be sent to Ireland in as large numbers as possible, and as early as the industrial situation in Britain admits." Some politicians regarded the labor movement as part of "the cataract of world events" sweeping the globe, as Churchill described it in imagery consistent with the concerns of flooding of boundaries and overwhelming of defenses we have seen in the last two chapters, seeing in nationalist movements in India and Ireland the hand of bolsheviks, who had infiltrated unions and the Labour party itself. Wilson repeatedly proclaimed to anyone who would listen that losing Ireland would mean losing India; losing the empire, he said, it would be only a matter of time before socialist revolution took hold. He warned that if the government did not take a stronger stand in Ireland the Irish question will be so complicated with the Labour question in England that it will become insoluble, and this would mean the loss of Ireland to begin with; the loss of the Empire in the second place; and the loss of England to finish up with. I have not been so nervous about the state of affairs in regard to the British Empire since July 1914,

he allowed, "and in many ways I am more anxious today than I was that fateful month."[43]

Labour leaders worried that the experiences of the police and soldiers in Ireland would redound negatively against workers at home. The Labour Commission report expressed concern about soldiers in Ireland who had had no training and displayed little discipline, "youths who at the most receptive period of their lives have been brutalized and demoralized." It especially marked out the Auxiliary Division of RIC as problematic. "This division is essentially undemocratic in its composition," it asserted. "It is a class weapon which is being forged in Ireland and could be used in England," a conclusion bolstered by a circular issued by the Royal Irish Constabulary after the publication of the commission's criticisms of Black and Tan atrocities. "We will remember this when next you go out on strike," it threatened.[44]

These concerns were not simply the fear-mongering of alarmist or opportunist labor leaders: Macready shared their anxieties. He confessed to Wilson,

I was thinking last night what would happen supposing some of these battalions were over in England a year or two hence and were called out in aid of Civil Power in a bad strike . . . . frankly I believe that troops who have been accustomed to reprising in this country would break loose if they had to face the conditions we had at Tonypandy, and if they did, no one knows better than you do what the results would be, both for the country, and to the Government of the day. This is the one thing that is worrying me very much.[45]

As it turned out, it was not the bloodymindedness of the troops he needed to worry about.

5
The General Strike of 1926

> Trade unions...must know perfectly well that in a general strike they will have the nation against them. Indignation and resentment are general among the body of the people at this attempt to force them into surrender. They will not surrender, and the sooner enemies of the people realize that they will not surrender, the better for them and for us all.[1]

The General Strike of 1926, which was described by contemporaries as "the greatest tragedy in the public, social and economic life of this country for the past century," commenced on 4 May, after negotiations to resolve a dispute between coal owners and coal miners over wages and hours broke down. Britons awoke on Tuesday, 4 May to an eerie and unprecedented silence. "A breathless feeling of intense quietness" prevailed, observed one Londoner, "such as comes before a thunderstorm." For, much to the surprise of the government and even of the Trades Union Congress (TUC), workers responded to the strike call with near-perfect solidarity. Public transport in London and other cities ceased almost completely: of the London Underground's 315 trains, 15 of them ran, and those only for short trips; all 4000 buses run by the London General Omnibus Company remained in their yards. The railroads halted and the docks sat idle. Starting around 8:00 A.M. commuters began their treks to work; on bicycles, on foot, in pony carts and traps, and in the backseats of tens of thousands of private automobiles, Britons made their way to their places of employment. "The first thing in the morning we stand at the window & watch the traffic in Southampton Row," Virginia Woolf recounted in her diary. "This is incessant. Everyone is bicycling; motor cars are huddled up with extra people. There are no buses. No placards. No newspapers. The men are at work in the road; water, gas & electricity are allowed; but at 11 the light was turned off." Traffic jams blocked virtually all the main arteries into London and streets clogged with vehicles that had come to a standstill. "From Marble Arch to Piccadilly," wrote Julian Symons, "traffic moved at only a few yards an hour, and on the Embankment...there was at times a solid block from Blackfriars to Westminster." The country had been shut down, and as Woolf lamented, "one does not know what to do."[2]

Britons had not received much warning; only on 3 May did they realize that a possible strike loomed. The TUC had committed itself to a general strike in support of the miners in late April, and called out its members when Baldwin's government announced the end of discussions designed to avoid a strike through a compromise settlement. Some 2.5 million workers answered the call that first day, halting coal production, shutting down the railways and public transportation, hampering commerce on the docks, restricting newspaper publication, and stopping delivery of the mail. For nine days, the strike continued to disrupt British economic life, but owing to the government's preparations for it; its access to public broadcasting through the BBC; the increased number of automobiles in private hands; the willingness of broad sections of the public to volunteer their time, efforts, and resources to keep things running; and, above all, the unwillingness of the unions to bring Britain to its knees by blocking distribution of food, fuel, and other vital necessities, the TUC called off the strike without having secured its aims. Coal miners stayed out for another six months, but they, too, capitulated without gaining the wage and hours agreement they had sought.

The trades unions and the Labour party regarded the General Strike as an industrial dispute, a characterization rejected by Conservative and Liberal politicians, newspapers, and interest groups who demonized unionized workers by painting the Labour party and unions as pawns of the bolshevik government in Russia. These groups portrayed the General Strike as a revolution, an assault on the institutions of parliamentary government, and a war against the British people.[3]

Fears and depictions of a revolutionary working class emerged immediately after the end of the war, fuelled—in the context of the Russian revolution and subsequent socialist risings in Europe—by soldier and worker unrest in early 1919 that seemed to threaten revolt in Britain. Strikes occurred with disconcerting regularity throughout 1919 and 1920, culminating in the spring of 1921 with a thwarted general strike. The first of these took place on the Clydeside in Glasgow in late January and February 1919, where, in "the battle of George Square," workers—some of them carrying the red flag of revolution—were confronted and set upon by police wielding batons. When the workers fought back, troops that had been waiting outside Glasgow with tanks and machine guns moved in and established order. A strike of the railwaymen followed in September 1919; when it threatened to turn into a general strike at the hands of the Triple Alliance of railwaymen, transport workers, and coal miners, Lloyd George's government intervened to settle the strike on the side of the workers. Eight months later, in May 1920, the London dock workers refused to load ships bound for Poland with arms intended to be used against Russia. In August, when the labor unions and the Labour party promised to shut down all of industry if Britain persisted in its efforts to intervene, the government capitulated. The earlier strikes, however frightening, had involved traditional wage demands; these latter actions were clearly political in nature.[4]

A final strike threat materialized in April 1921, after a three-month period in which unemployment doubled. When the government announced that it would abdicate its wartime controls over the coal mines, mine owners declared their intention to reduce wage rates and return to the prewar system of paying wages on the basis of pit production, a policy that would negatively affect those who worked inefficient or inferior mines. Miners demanded instead the continuance of equalized rates across the mines, which owners answered with a lockout. The Triple Alliance called a general strike for 1 April 1921, but before it could begin the railwaymen and transport workers chose to continue negotiations with the government, betraying, in the eyes of the miners, labor solidarity. The government had averted a general strike on "Black Friday," as embittered workers called it, but could not be sanguine that another would not break out. The sense of class conflict and animosity toward workers approached dangerous levels: as Richard Aldington observed, "this interminable series of strikes and lockouts looked remarkably like warfare." Indeed, battalions that might have gone to Ireland to repress the IRA could not be spared, for fear that they would be needed at home to contend with striking workers. In April 1921, Lloyd George's cabinet had discussed how many troops would be necessary for "holding the British coalfields," as Neville Chamberlain put it. Secretary of War Lamington Worthington-Evans declared that "we need 18 battalions to hold London," and proposed taking two of them from Malta, four from the Rhine, and one or two from Egypt. Henry Wilson suggested that "loyal citizens could join the territorials" in defending London, in particular, taking which, Lloyd George agreed, would be "the important thing in a revolutionary movement."[5]

Fears of worker revolution figured prominently in postwar politics. After the armistice, Conservatives had agreed to continue in Lloyd George's wartime coalition government because they could not be sure that the newly enfranchised working classes would not decimate their ranks at the polls. The Coalition, it seemed to them and to Liberals as well, appeared to offer the strongest bulwark against the mass of returning soldiers whose attitudes were unknown and actions unpredictable. Despite the very vocal misgivings of Die-Hard Conservatives, who, at the 1920 conference of the National Union of Conservative and Unionist Associations, castigated Lloyd George for having "hobnobbed with Bolsheviks" and charged that Labour's program of nationalization would result in "the nationalisation of women." Coalition Conservatives like Austen Chamberlain persuaded the bulk of the party, which had not won a general election since 1900, that the Coalition, representing "a great middle body of opinion," was best positioned to address the political, social, and economic changes wrought by the war, and in so doing, stave off the threat of revolution. Offering increased educational opportunities, housing, unemployment payments, and, in 1921, "uncovenanted benefits" to those not making contributions to the unemployment fund seemed to Coalition members to provide, as Lloyd George put it, "a cheap insurance against Bolshevism." When they grumbled about the "socialistic" nature of these expenditures, Chamberlain cautioned restive Conservatives that dissolution of the Coalition government could result in "breaking the forces of order."[6]

The measures instituted to absorb unemployed soldiers and fend off revolution caused inflation, disgruntling an increasing number of middle-class men and women whose fixed incomes limited their ability to cope with rising prices. Seeing workers making gains at their expense, these voters turned in droves to the Conservative party. In the early 1920s, Conservatives increased their membership dramatically to some 700,000, twice the membership enjoyed by the Labour party; much of that increase came from the middle-class suburbs. Organized in grass-roots interest groups such as the Anti-Waste League and the Middle-Class Union and given voice by newspapers such as the *Daily Express* and the *Daily Mail*, the largest mass-circulation dailies throughout the 1920s, middle-class voters made their discontent with the Coalition known, forcing the establishment, in 1922, of the Geddes committee, which was charged with identifying areas of public expenditure that could be reduced. The committee's diligence produced deep cuts in the budget for education, housing, and the military.

Conservative successes derived from the party's ability to cast workers as "a unionized working class with whom [the middle classes] were perpetually in conflict and for whose greed they would have to pay." These stereotypes helped to forge a consciousness among a vast body of middle-class Britons who perceived themselves to be the "constitutional classes," the loyal bulwark standing between the country and ruin brought about by an aggressive, unionized working class. It was these people, argues Ross McKibbin, "whose loyalty to the government during the general strike [of 1926] was as intense as the solidarity of the strikers." As E.H.H. Green has noted, "if the Great War and the immediate post-war period saw a rise in 'class consciousness,' this was as much a trend in middle-class social and political life as it was in the much more extensively studied world of working-class life, labour, and politics."[7]

By the summer of 1922, displeasure with Coalition Conservatives had grown sufficiently that the party could no longer hold out; it voted to secede from Lloyd George's coalition government and forced a new election. Baldwin explained that Conservatives must abandon the Coalition and return to the partisan ways of the past because the very existence of the party depended upon it. Using the imagery of shattering that we have seen operating in so many areas of life, he warned that the "dynamic force" of Lloyd George, which had "smashed to pieces" the Liberal party, threatened to do the same to Conservatives. "I think if the present association is continued . . . you will see . . . the old Conservative Party . . . smashed to atoms and lost in ruins . . . by the disintegrating influence of a dynamic force."[8]

The unity of the party derived from its implacable opposition to socialism, a terrifying, if amorphous, enemy in which were lumped not just bolsheviks and communists, but trade unionists, the TUC, and the Labour party as well. Its effectiveness in mobilizing primitive fears and prejudices can be seen in its polling: McKibbin estimates that the Conservative party received a majority of working-class votes in the 1920s. Only the presence of the Liberal candidates, who siphoned off votes that would almost certainly have gone to the Tories, gave the 1923 election to the Labour party.[9]

Labour's victory rocked conservatives of all stripes. Churchill regarded it as "a serious national misfortune such as has usually befallen great States only on the morrow of defeat in war." Unprepared for power and unaccustomed to the responsibility of governing, Labour foundered over the issue of normalizing relations with Russia, and Prime Minister Ramsay MacDonald was forced to call an election in October 1924. One of the dirtiest campaigns ever fought, the election of 1924 centered on the question of Labour's affiliation, as Conservatives and Liberals saw it, with the bolshevik government of Russia. Joynson-Hicks, who would become Home Secretary in Baldwin's government, referred, in *The Times* of 12 April 1924, to MacDonald's government as "interlopers." In May, he declared that "at the next General Election...the whole burden of the contest with revolutionary Socialism will fall upon the Conservative Party." He warned Liberal voters that they had to decide whether they were for the "Constitution or Labour which was against the Constitution," urging them to cast their votes for the Conservative party, lest the contests in the three-party constituencies produce a victory for Labour MPs. Labour, Conservative party literature declared, was not above passing off communist spies as health visitors or enticing children to Sunday schools where communists would brainwash them and teach them how to carry out street fighting; resurrecting the alarms of the 1920 NUCA conference, Conservatives claimed that communist aims to nationalize social and economic institutions promised to destroy marriage and the family by nationalizing women. The one communist in the election contest, Shapurji Saklatvala, an Indian seeking to represent Battersea, was described by the *Daily Express* in now familiar imagery as "a little dark skinned" man whose oratory reminded the writer of "a great cataract of words always spouting, frothing, foaming from him in a never-ending stream."[10]

Stanley Baldwin, whose reputation for moderation and compromise has been overstated, did not shy away from embracing this kind of demonizing language against Labour; and, like Joynson-Hicks and other Conservative party campaigners, he leavened his speeches with healthy doses of anti-alien, anti-Semitic rhetoric. In his 16 October 1924 broadcast, Baldwin alluded to the unrest evident in Britain in association with his denunciation of "alien" subversives. "We cannot afford the luxury of academic socialists or revolutionary agitation," he declared over the airways. "I think it's high time somebody said to Russia 'Hands off England.' " He then promised that as Prime Minister he would "examine the laws and regulations as to the entry of aliens into this country, for in these days no alien should be substituted for one of our own people when we have not enough work at home to go around." *The Times*, on 24 October, carried a story headlined "SOVIET SHIP AT PORT TALBOT, Communists in Close Touch with Crew." Port Talbot was located within MacDonald's constituency, and the paper used this fact to suggest that Liberals stumping in the area had encountered "serious interruption when they referred to the Russian Treaty." The rhetoric and representation of Labour as socialist, and socialists as communists, and communists as bolsheviks operated to portray Labour party members and union members as a non-British, alien presence, complete with "long hair, bulging eyes, squat noses, bristling moustaches and scrubbing-brush beards. It was the image of a 'stage Cossack,' " noted Anne Perkins. These very images populated the pages of the popular press.[11]

All of this prepared the way for the "discovery," on 25 October, just days before the 1924 election, of a letter to British communists, purporting to come from Grigory Zinoviev, Russian President of the Third International, characterizing MacDonald's efforts to normalize relations with Russia as support for the revolution; he also, allegedly, commanded the British communist party to infiltrate the military forces with an eye to fomenting mutiny among them. The so-called Zinoviev letter, which the Conservative party's central office made available to the *Daily Mail* for publication, virtually guaranteed Labour's defeat. Conservatives used the Zinoviev letter to cast the Labour party—and MacDonald in particular—as the enemy of the British people. On the day the *Daily Mail* published the letter, Lord Birkenhead issued a blast against the "class hatred" preached by socialists, which, he averred, "is alien to our soil." He reminded readers that during the war, "when the honour of the country was at stake, men of all classes, rich and poor alike, rallied to the colours." There were exceptions, he added, to this very British display of patriotism, "some men who let their fellows go and themselves stayed behind," often at the encouragement of men like Ramsay MacDonald. "You will find," Birkenhead promised, "that it is precisely among these men that the loudest preachers of class hatred are to be found to-day."[12] The *Mail*'s editorial that day followed with the announcement that Zinoviev's call for the infiltration of the army by British communists was but a prelude to "a great outbreak of the abominable 'class war,' which is civil war of the most savage kind. Preparations are to be pressed forward in England for 'an armed insurrection,' " the paper informed readers, implicating Labour in the plot. Insisting that the "Socialist Government" of Ramsay MacDonald "is under the control of the Communist Party," the *Mail* charged Labour with doing "the bidding of the murderous, alien despotism in Moscow." The Prime Minister, it declared, "is betraying the British nation," "plotting the utter ruin of this country."[13] Like Birkenhead, the paper reminded readers that when the war broke out in 1914, MacDonald showed his true, treacherous colors by accusing the Admiralty of fomenting war in order "to give the Navy 'battle-practice.' "[14] These references to the war continued throughout the week, providing a context of national danger within which MacDonald's purported betrayal of the country could be heightened. Birkenhead warned Conservative voters that should any stay away from the polls he would be "deserting his country in the hour of the greatest peril it has known since 1914. Your sons, fathers and husbands did not fail then," he proclaimed. "Will you fail now?" MacDonald, "our shifty Prime Minister," he called him, invoking the classic imagery of the Eastern European Jew, had failed his country in 1914; should Conservative voters stay at home, "you are false to your dead."[15] They did not, and were not, returning a majority of 207 Conservatives to the House. The election, claimed the *Mail*, which saw "The Red Flag Blown to Shreds," had saved Britain.[16]

Returning to power in 1924, many Conservatives continued to portray unionists and Labour party members as socialists, often conflating socialists, communists, and bolsheviks. Baldwin, having secured office for himself and his party, reverted to a conciliatory tone and tried to check some of his colleagues' excesses, as when the party sought to eliminate provisions allowing trade unions to use member dues for political activity. "We stand for peace," he told his followers.

> We want to create an atmosphere, a new atmosphere in a new Parliament for a new age, in which the people can come together . . . I know that there are those who work for different ends from most of us in this House, yet there are many in all ranks and all parties who will re-echo my prayer: 'Give peace in our time, O Lord.'

Despite his efforts, Conservatives—and sometimes Baldwin himself—persisted in regarding and representing to the country the image of Labour and trade unionists as enemies of the nation.[17]

In the spring of 1925, coal miners threatened to strike again over the owners' efforts to cut wages and increase hours. The owners stood firm, refusing to concede any ground; a strike was averted only when the government agreed to provide a stipend to the industry that would ensure the status quo for a year, to the end of April 1926. For the next year, Conservative politicians and newspaper editors conducted a loud and incessant campaign against the purported threat of a communist rising. Joynson-Hicks warned, "the thing is not finished. The danger is not over. Is England to be governed by Parliament or by a handful of trade union leaders? If a Soviet is established here . . . a grave position will arise." In a speech in Battersea, Churchill insisted that "behind Socialism stands Communism. Behind Communism, Moscow, that dark sinister evil power, a band of cosmopolitan conspirators." MacDonald and other politicians tried to refute charges that Labour ranks included significant numbers of communists, MacDonald castigating the Conservative party for its "wanton use of Communism for purely party purposes." At the Labour party conference in the fall of 1925, delegates voted to refuse membership to communists. These efforts did little to still the attacks on the party. In April 1926, for instance, Lieutenant-Colonel Sir Alan Burgoyne introduced a motion in the House of Commons

> That, in the opinion of this House, rigorous measures should be taken to suppress the revolutionary propaganda which is being carried on in Great Britain and the Empire, both amongst the civil population and the armed forces of the Crown, by organisations which have for their object the overthrow of the British Constitution.

In no uncertain terms, he laid that propagandizing at the feet of the Labour party. "The party opposite are by no means guiltless in helping this propaganda to dive deep into the body of our nation." "Right hon. Gentlemen opposite who sit on the Labour benches have associated themselves with the Communist movement." He dismissed Labour's efforts to distance the party from communism, their "great parade of turning out the Communists" through "pious resolutions passed at packed party meetings," as mere show. "They condemn it in public, they cherish it in secret.... They throw it out, but they come back to it again as a dog returns to its vomit." Lietuenant-Commander Kenworthy protested that "this cry of Communist propaganda" was leading "people in other countries... to... think we are on the verge of a revolution. Everyone knows that the institutions of this country have never been more stable and that we have never been further from a revolution than at the present time." His words fell on deaf ears.[18]

Many contemporaries and subsequent historians have regarded the government's willingness to provide a subsidy to the coal industry as a means of buying time that would enable it to prepare for a general strike that it saw coming but was not then, in 1925, ready to counter. Indeed, under the leadership of Joynson-Hicks at the Home Office, the government began secretly to lay plans. Baldwin noted that if a strike occurred, the "community has to protect itself, with the full strength of the Government behind it, the community will do so, and the response of the community will astonish the forces of anarchy throughout the world." Joynson-Hicks chaired the Supply and Transport Committee, an emergency agency charged with recruiting and coordinating volunteers to help keep services running in the event of a strike. J.C.C. Davidson was named Chief Civil Commissioner and given the responsibility of planning for the possibility of revolution. He appointed a number of military men to posts as deputy civil commissioners with the charge of organizing and recruiting throughout the country. So great did popular fears of worker revolution become in consequence of endless alarms raised by politicians and the press that Baldwin felt it necessary to allay those concerns by announcing Davidson's strike plans in November 1925. Under the Emergency Powers Act of 1920, the government had the right to seize property; appropriate food, water, and medicines; commandeer private transport; and take control of the docks, railways, coal and oil supplies, and all public utilities. It could prohibit meetings and issue orders for searches of premises. Separate from the government's preparations, a volunteer Organization for the Maintenance of Supplies (OMS) had formed in September 1925, with the object of registering volunteers who would help "defeat the Communist conspiracy" and "provide a defense against the Reds." In a recruitment poster for the York branch of the OMS, the Thirsk and Malton Conservative Association declared that strikers would overthrow the current government and set up one "chosen by a revolutionary element composed of aliens!"[19] Amongst the volunteers to the OMS, Joynson-Hicks made clear in a letter to Baldwin, were the British Fascists: "they are well known," he asserted, "and, I think to be depended upon. I have seen their leaders many times." Baldwin appears to have accepted this piece of information without comment. The Home Office was careful to prevent "organised" bodies of fascists from enlisting as special constables under the emergency plan, but as one of its officials explained, "as specials, working individually under the orders of the police, they should be eligible recruits." Cabinet officials were informed in October 1925 that in addition to the OMS, the "Fascisti . . . would, in the case of an emergency, be at the disposal of the Government."[20]

By the time the 1925 coal subsidy was due to expire, the government was ready. Baldwin negotiated for three days with the leadership of the Labour party and that of the TUC in order to find a solution, but, pushed by members of his cabinet such as Neville Chamberlain, Churchill, and Joynson-Hicks, who thought he needed "firming up" in the face of a menace that must be met head on and defeated, he abruptly broke off talks on 3 May. Strike notices that had gone out earlier in the event of a breakdown in negotiations were confirmed by telegraph, and the strike officially began at midnight on the third. Baldwin told the House of Commons that the government had stopped negotiations because "it found itself challenged with an alternative Government." The Labour party and the unions, he insisted, were "entering on a course which, if successful on the part of those who enter on it, can only substitute tyranny. It is not wages that are imperilled; it is the freedom of our very Constitution." In language reminiscent of those recalling their state of mind during the war, he told the House that "everything that I care for is being smashed to bits at this moment," but promised that "I shall pick up the bits.... we shall pass, after much suffering, through deep waters and through storms, to that better land for which we hope." Churchill, far more strident than Baldwin in his characterization of the strike, set the tone for the government and for much of the rest of the country as well. He declared that the unions had instigated "a conflict which, if it is fought out to a conclusion, can only end in the overthrow of Parliamentary Government or in its decisive victory," insisting that the country could demand no less than unconditional surrender of the unions. "There is no middle course open," he asserted.

> Either the Parliamentary institutions of the country will emerge tri-umphant, and the nation, which has not flinched in the past through many ordeals, the nation, which indeed has always shown itself stronger and nobler and more generous in its hours of trouble, will once again maintain itself and be mistress in its own house, or else, on the other hand, the existing constitution will be fatally injured, and.... the consequences of their action will inevitably lead to the erection of some Soviet of trade unions on which, whether under Parliamentary forms or without them, the real effective control of the economic and political life of the country will devolve.... we are bound to face this present challenge unflinchingly, rigorously, rigidly, and resolutely to the end.[21]

Language like this echoed that mobilized during the Great War to invigorate Britons in their fight against the German Hun. Indeed, analogies to the Great War permeated public discourse and peppered private conversation as well. Liberal Sir John Simon explained to the House that "we speak of this situation as a 'general strike' much in the same way as we speak of the last war as the 'great war,' because it is something of exceptional gravity and importance and suffering." In a 11 May 1926 speech, he virtually conflated striking workers with the German enemy of 1914–1918, reminding his colleagues of

> what it was like when the Germans tried to bomb London from Zeppelins. The Germans knew so little of the British character that

they thought that, by putting people living in London to inconve- nience or it might be to danger, they would somehow advance their cause. I never could have believed that any countrymen of mine, who know the British character as well as any of us do, and who are just as good specimens of the British character as any of us, would have thought that you could possibly secure public support for their cause by operations which are designed to put inconvenience and possibly danger upon the general inhabitants of this land.

"This thing is a war," he insisted.[22]

Led by the example of Baldwin, Churchill, Joynson-Hicks, and Simon, other politicians and newspaper editors dismissed the General Strike as an industrial action on behalf of higher wages and depicted it as an attack on the nation. In an editorial entitled "Our Duty," *The Times* denounced "the bitter trial of a general strike" that had been "wan- tonly thrust upon us." It expressed confidence that the British people would "'keep steady' whatever happens, as steady as they kept during the worst days of the war. Foolish and provocative speeches will not tempt them into indiscretions any more than did the exasperating lan- guage of 'pacifists' and 'defeatists' in the deadly struggle with Germany." "Trade unions...must know perfectly well that in a general strike they will have the nation against them," it warned. "Indignation and resent- ment are general among the body of the people at this attempt to force them into surrender. They will not surrender, and the sooner enemies of the people realize that they will not surrender, the better for them and for us all." Sir Robert Horne declared in the House that "there was no episode in the war which created so much anxiety and apprehension in our breasts as the thought that those who would ordinarily be acting with us are determined to ally themselves against the Government at this stage," but promised that "the whole instincts of the British peo- ple will revolt against any attempt to take from them their freedom and plant tyranny in place of constitutional Government."[23]

We might regard these efforts to cast the strike as equivalent to the Great War, and strikers as equivalent to the German enemy, as a bid to eliminate unionized workers from "the nation." Certainly, these speeches and editorials intensified the sense of a military conflict between striking workers and the rest of the country. The *British Gazette*, the government's official newspaper edited by Churchill from the offices of the *Morning Post*, carried a message from Henry Asquith on 8 May under the banner, "British People on the Rack. Strike Weapon Aimed at Daily Life of the Community. Must be Sheathed Before Negotiations."

Asquith was reported to have said that the strike was not an industrial action, but aimed to substitute a "Dictatorship" for "Free Government." *The Times* called the strike

> the gravest domestic menace which has hung over this nation since the fall of the Stuarts...The leaders declare earnestly, and no doubt sincerely, that they have not any quarrel with the people and are not declaring war upon them; but the assertion will not bear the test of the plain facts.

In subsequent editorials throughout the strike it referred frequently to "the menace to the national life and to the Constitution," characterizing the strike by turns "an immeasurable danger," a "disaster...to the whole nation"[24]

The *Daily Mail* in an editorial entitled "For King and Country!" called the strike

> a revolutionary movement intended to inflict suffering upon the great mass of innocent persons in the community and thereby to put forcible constraint upon the Government. It is a movement which can only succeed by destroying the government and subverting the rights and liberties of the people.... it must be dealt with by every resource at the disposal of the community.

On the first day of the strike, it accused MacDonald of leading "this attempt to coerce the community and terrorise the Government." "There are now two Governments in this country," the paper insisted, establishing a showdown between His Majesty's government and that of the TUC. "Two Governments cannot exist in the same capital. The one must destroy the other or surrender to the other."[25]

This rhetoric of war corresponded with the government's determination to meet the strike with a quasi-military response. Hyde Park became the government's strategic distribution center for milk and food. Looking for all the world like an army encampment, with tents, huts, generators, and utility lines running through it, the park provided a base for the railway companies and served as the depot for buses and lorries. Thousands of volunteers congregated here as they awaited their assignments, serviced by canteens, rest areas, recreation rooms, and toilet facilities. Men in khaki uniforms, special constables wearing helmets, armed soldiers and sailors, mounted police, and armored cars patrolled the streets and guarded power stations and the docks. Sentries at Buckingham Palace and other royal residences donned service khaki.

(Outside of London, Davidson's civil commissioners handled the distribution of food and fuel with less visible displays of strike-breaking.) In the early morning of day five of the strike, a long convoy of lorries accompanied by armored cars filled with armed soldiers made its way to the East End in order to open the docks. Observers would have seen "guardsmen," as Perkin described them, "wearing the same uniform they had worn on the battlefields of Europe less than ten years earlier, steel helmets and grey greatcoats and, at the controls, Tank Corps soldiers in their distinctive black caps," making their way through Bow and Poplar, areas, as Perkins reminds us, that to much of Britain, "were a foreign country." Joynson-Hicks reportedly told army commanders that the opening of the docks justified virtually any amount of armed force; certainly the *British Gazette* and the *Daily Express* of 8 May carried the announcement by the government that "All ranks—the armed forces of the Crown—are hereby notified that any action they may find it necessary to take in an honest endeavour to aid the civil power will receive both now and afterwards the full support of HM Government." The government's display of military force continued throughout the strike, even when it appeared to be at its end: Virginia Woolf reported in her diary on the last day of the strike that she had seen, that morning, "5 or 6 armoured cars slowly going along Oxford Street; on each two soldiers sat in tin helmets, & one stood with his hand at the gun which was pointed straight ahead, ready to fire." When she tried to convey to her sister Vanessa what life was like in London during the strike, she could not. "It beggars description," she despaired in a letter, except to "recall the worst days of the war."[26]

From the start, rumors of violence, mutiny, and insurrection fuelled the military atmosphere. The *Daily Mail*'s 3 May issue blared, "Troops on the Move."

A battalion of the Cheshire Regiment arrived at Cardiff yesterday. This is one of the troop movements which the Government has ordered as a precautionary measure. Detachments are also being moved into Lancashire and Scotland in order to be available, should the necessity arise, to assist the police in the maintenance of law and order and the protection of life and property. The 5th Infantry Brigade at Aldershot, comprising several thousand troops, are standing ready to proceed north. Nearly a mile of motor-coaches and transport wagons were in readiness last night to convey the troops to their destination. Iron rations have been issued for a three-day period. All arms are standing by, and men have been recalled from leave.

The 6 May issue carried headlines like: "5,000 Strikers Rush Police. Defence with Truncheons." "East-End Disorders. Four Motor-Cars Burned." "Volunteers Attacked. Police Protect Tramcar Services." "Warship Movements." "Troops at Smithfield." "Steel Helmet 'Specials.' Government Create Full-Time Force." "Shops Looted at Hull. Sailors Out with Fixed Bayonets." "Collision in a Tunnel. Two Killed & Seven Injured. Police and Soldiers Gassed." (This last headline was typically misstated: the men had been overcome when a gas tank was dislodged in a collision between a train and a motor car.) The *British Gazette* proclaimed to readers on 7 May 1926, "Strikers Attack Police. Windows of Tramcars Smashed." Then, in smaller type, "No Serious Injury." The next day, it warned Britons of an "Organised Attempt to Starve the Nation.... Situation Becoming More Intense." *The Times* was no less shrill in its coverage, informing readers that "an organised attempt is being made to starve the people and to wreck the State." "Riotous Scenes in Scotland," it reported. "Edinburgh Shops Looted," "Baton Charge at Hull," "Police Attacked with Bottles," "Threats with Revolver," "More Rioting in Glasgow. Prolonged Fights with Police," "Rioting at Hull," ran the headlines.[27]

Joynson-Hicks's call, on the first day of the strike, for 30,000 special constables heightened the sense of communal warfare, leading people like Arnold Bennett and Sidney Webb to fear the worst. Bennett noted in his diary on the second day of the strike the "general opinion that the fight would be short but violent. Bloodshed anticipated next week." Webb told his wife Beatrice that he was "far more apprehensive of a long strike and bloodshed in the streets before it ended." He impressed upon her his belief that "the working-class generally is far more anxious to strike than the...T.U.C. and that in certain industrial areas—Newcastle and Glasgow—there is a very ugly spirit which, if the stoppage continued and there were hunger, might mean outbursts of violence between the workers and the police." The War Office placed its security branch, MI5, on alert, and went so far as to send soldiers in mufti to infiltrate pubs in the East End in order to keep watch on the civilian population. On day four, Joynson-Hicks called for 50,000 more special constables; the following day, the government announced the establishment of a new police force in London, the Civil Constabulary Reserve, comprised of full-time volunteers recruited from the Territorial forces and Officer Training Corps and commanded by Sir Neville Macready, who, the *Daily Mail* reminded its readers, "was Commander-in-Chief in Ireland during the troublous period." Men like C.H. Drage, a naval officer, responded immediately. He was assigned to the U.C. division at the Admirality. "U.C. stands for Unrest, Civil," he explained in his journal. "The Section was working at top pressure and expanding at the same time. At noon a parcel of 12 service pistols were brought in by an old Admiralty messenger—so now we can defend ourselves." The *British Gazette* assured volunteers on 5 May 1926 that "special constables who are injured in the execution of their duty, and widows and children in case of death, will be granted pensions allowances or gratuities." These were, of course, the kind of benefits granted to the families of soldiers and sailors who fought in the Great War.[28]

Prepped for years for the prospect of communist revolution, significant portions of British society responded to the unions' actions as if they were a war against their institutions and way of life. Goaded by politicians and the press, many Britons had internalized the view of unionized workers as enemies; after the alarms raised by Joynson-Hicks and Churchill of the prospects of violence and bloodshed, they prepared, many of them, for combat. Margaret Woods, aged about 15, wrote in her diary on day four,

> Dad is splendid in the strike. He takes up people every morning and keeps a weapon on the seat beside him, because many of the Bolshy roughs like to demonstrate their feelings on the hardworking citizens and their doins is not [sic] by any means pleasant. People are all well protected though by police and special constables and riots have been quickly suppressed by baton charges.

Henry Duckworth, part of a contingent of Cambridge men who packed off to Dover to help keep the port open, kept a diary of those days. His 6 May entry refers to the students as "troops," giving a hint as to the frame of mind of his companions. "Numerous rumours were about as to the strikers' attitude towards us," he reported. "It was thought that there might be a massed attack on us during the night." On 7 May,

> a message was brought to us that 500 strikers were on their way up to the station to storm us.... Everyone was armed to the teeth with pieces of lead piping, spanners and other equally effective weapons.... But everything remained quiet and peaceful and shortly after midnight everyone was able to return to rest.

The next night, 8 May, Duckworth noted that "shortly after eleven we were informed that four hundred men were on the way up to murder us.... everyone went to their allotted positions.... a few of the reported army turned up, but their numbers were certainly not more than forty" and were handled by the local police with little to-do. The nightly alarms unnerved the Cambridge students, despite their protests that they sought armed protection during the night only so that they might get a full night's sleep and be prepared for a hard day's work on the morrow; ultimately, "a special gang was formed of some of the strongest members of the party to become Special Constables."[29]

Although actual violence, as opposed to the rumors spread by newspapers and word of mouth, remained relatively contained, it did take place, and frequently enough to concern union and Labour leaders. Strikers' attempts to keep volunteers from running public transport led to police baton charges in Glasgow, Leeds, Doncaster, London, and many other cities and towns in Scotland and the north of England. Davidson confided that in Leeds "the Chief Constable broke 32 truncheons and a vast number of the right heads the first night of the strike."[30] "Special constables were acquiring a rough reputation," observed Perkins, "and they were often accused of provoking or aggravating strikers and pickets." She wrote of

a determined chief constable [in Brighton] who... decided to recruit mounted specials. A trio of local cavalry officers, two retired and one on leave from India, each raised an assorted troop of men from the farms and villages of the surrounding area, who were sworn in and issued with two batons, one short and one long, 'for use in charges.' They called themselves the Black and Tans after the regiment notorious for its brutal treatment of the Irish.

MP Haden Guest expressed his concern to the House of Commons on 10 May 1926 about police reprisals being carried out against his constituency: "That is a policy of what used to be called in the bad days of Ireland a policy of reprisals. It led to a terrible tragedy in that country. I hope it is not going to reopen a chapter of such tragedy in this country."[31]

Trade unionists, Labour leaders, and their allies tried in vain to counter their depiction as revolutionaries or enemies of the people and to present workers as full and responsible citizens of the nation. J.H. Thomas protested to the House on 3 May that contrary to the cabinet's representations of strikers as threats to the British way of life, "this course was taken, not by anti-patriots, not by people who wanted a revolution, not by people who do not love their country, not by people who desired an upheaval." Workers, he insisted, far from being the enemies of society, were "trustees for the nation." Picking up on his language, the *Daily Herald* called upon Stanley Baldwin to "act as the trustee for the interests of the nation, and not as the head of a Party which exists to safeguard the interests of a few." "Let him be the Prime Minister of the People," the paper exhorted Baldwin, rather than the leader of those who believe they "represent the fine flower of the race, and are therefore entitled to the best of everything." Workers were acting in the interests of the country as a whole; the government, by contrast, the paper charged, "has considered not national, but class and party interests." Trades unionists had embarked upon an industrial action in a dispute with mine owners in order to preserve the hard-fought gains and well-being of a significant national constituency; they were, in fact, serving the national interest by doing so. "The men and women who are concerned in this strike...are part of the nation," protested MP Viant before the House of Commons on 7 May. "The Trades Union General Council is not making war on the people," insisted the *British Worker*. Rather, "it is anxious that the ordinary members of the public shall not be penalised for the unpatriotic conduct of the mineowners and the Government."[32]

In a "Message to all Workers" the TUC urged strikers to exhibit moderation and peaceableness in their actions so as "not to give any opportunity for police interference." Disturbances, the leadership feared, would make it difficult for strikers to succeed in their aims, not least because violence and disorder would play into the hands of those like Joynson-Hicks, whose "provocative utterances" and "inference...that the Trade Union Movement was violating law and order" were calculated to panic the public and to turn it against them. Strikers, far from engaging in insurrection, "mean to conduct themselves in a disciplined, quiet and orderly manner." There was, the *British Worker* insisted, "No Attack on the Constitution." "There is no Constitutional Crisis," it reiterated the next day. Not only, the paper reported, had local union leaders issued directives to their rank and file membership that "police orders shall be obeyed, and all disorder avoided," but strikers were going out of their way to cooperate with the police.

At Lewes the police and the strikers have organised a public billiards match, whilst the Forest of Dean police have received a letter from the local trade union organisation saying that union members are open to assist the police in maintaining order in any way which the police think fit.[33]

Union and Labour leaders tried to counter depictions of workers as enemies of the nation by playing up the war service given by so many of them; the *British Worker* observed that "as a reply to the perverted patriotism of Government supporters many of the striking transport and railway workers are wearing their war medals." If anything could establish them as members of the nation, it seemed, participation in the war should do it, and supporters of the strikers used every opportunity to remind the public of the great sacrifices they had made during the war. Sometimes, those sacrifices were trotted out to justify the demands of the miners, as when the *Daily Herald* said of the seven-hour day, "the whole Labour Movement values it as the fruit of a hard, long fight and a victory won. It was the chief instalment secured, out of so many promised and shabbily withheld, towards making Britain the Land Fit for Heroes, of which we heard during the war." More often, however, strike supporters referred to wartime service in order to shame the government and the mine owners for their treatment of workers. A letter to the *Daily Herald* from Richard Morris, formerly MP for Battersea, for example, noted that "many of the aggrieved workmen carry on their bodies the scars from enemy bullets, attested to by decorations from the King." He described those members of the printers' union who refused to print for the *Daily Mail* a "For King and Country" issue just before the onset of the strike as "men who, rightly or wrongly, considered themselves entitled to restrain the profane use of the banner under which they had fought." They should be regarded, he claimed, as men "who refused to be branded as traitors to their King and Country, with their battle wounds hardly healed." MP R. Morrison urged his colleagues to remember that

> these chaps who are walking about the streets to-day on strike are the same people who were in the Army from 1914 to 1918.... the same lads I marched along with on the other side, and they are showing the same capacity. Someone quoted on Saturday a famous German war *communiqué* issued at the time of the Battle of Amiens: 'The British are holding on with their usual tenacity.' That is exactly the position of these workers—holding on with their usual tenacity. They have not suddenly become scoundrels. They are perfectly honest and law-abiding citizens.

"These men who are out on strike to-day are the same fellows whom you patted on the back during the Great War," he reminded them. George Lansbury lamented the show of force the government was putting on against strikers, telling MPs that "I stood this morning in Bow Road and saw those great armoured cars trundling along the road." To the cheers of approval made by other MPs, he responded, "well, all right, that is the sort of terrorism that you are exercising against people in the part of London that sent more men in proportion to its population to the War than any other—this is the way you treat them under these conditions."[34]

The strike ended on 12 May, when the TUC capitulated to the government's demand for an unconditional surrender. Although he refused to negotiate any terms, Baldwin let union leaders believe that a memorandum of understanding worked out by Herbert Samuel could serve as a basis for a settlement. (In the event, the strikers got nothing but an undertaking by Baldwin that he would urge employers not to retaliate against them when they returned to work.) In a burst of misplaced self-congratulation, the *Daily Herald* carried a story by former editor George Lansbury entitled "Those Unforgettable Nine Days!" in which he compared the impact of the strike to that of the Great War. Just as the war had left no institution or person untouched, Lansbury argued, the strike had shaken British society to its core. With the advent of the war,

> the earth quaked; the pots were all jostled. Some were broken; some were cracked. They may be standing still, and to some eyes they may look unharmed, but they can never be as they were before. They would fall to pieces at the lightest blow. It will be found in the days which are coming that, in a smaller sphere, the General Strike has had the same effect.

If Lansbury thought the strike had weakened the government, he was sadly mistaken. Emergency powers that had been enacted on 1 May to meet the possibility of the strike were kept in place until the miners returned to work in December; they gave the government the continued right to use orders-in-council to set up summary courts and to take whatever actions it deemed necessary to keep essential supplies and functions up and running. The government took the opportunity presented by the strike to enact a series of policies Conservatives had long sought to impose: "vindictiveness has now seized our masters," Virginia Woolf noted in her diary. In the coal areas, where the miners were still out, Neville Chamberlain, as Minister of Health, used the newly passed Boards of Guardians (Default) Act to disband the elected boards of guardians and replace them with government-appointed commissioners. In such places as Bedwellty, the new commissioners slashed poor relief payments to families to less than a third of that paid to feed, clothe, and house residents of workhouses in the area.[35]

The government took advantage of labor's defeat to repeal the Eight Hours Act and to pass the Trades Disputes Act of 1927, which rendered general strikes illegal and punishable by two years in prison; changed the system of the political levy so vital to the existence of the Labour party so that workers had to agree to "contract in" rather than "contract out" of contributing to their unions' political funds; forbade civil servants and local government employees from new membership in unions with any TUC affiliation; and outlawed "intimidation" by strikers, which was broadly and vaguely enough defined as to mean almost anything. It certainly had the potential to make picketing employers much more difficult. As historians have pointed out, the terms of the act were rarely invoked, and had little material impact on the labor movement, though Labour party coffers certainly declined dramatically over the next few years, in some estimations by as much as a quarter. But as a symbolic measure of workers' defeat at the hands of "the nation" it held great significance, and even Churchill's wartime coalition government refused to repeal it (only when Labour came to power in 1946 was the hated act done away with). One ironic effect of Conservatives' efforts to kick their opponents when they were down, to make them "lick it," as the Manchester *Guardian* put it, was a resurgence of Labour party votes in the 1929 election, bringing to power for a short-lived reign the second MacDonald government of the decade.[36]

If the strike, to use Lansbury's words, had left any institution so shaken that it "would fall to pieces at the lightest blow," it appeared to be the trade union movement itself. C.F.G. Masterson, continuing the theme of fracturing that we have seen characterizing the experience of the war, wrote in the *Contemporary Review*, "suddenly the strike cracked and broke in a manner that resembled nothing so much as the cracking and breaking of the German armies in the autumn of 1918." "The trade union world lies shattered and in ruins," he asserted, employing the now familiar imagery of wartime. Union membership declined from 5.2 million to 4.8 million between 1926 and 1928. The number of days lost to strikes fell from 162 million in 1926 to 1.2 million in 1927 and 1.4 million in 1928. Certainly, the miners lost out completely: their holdout produced no concessions. In fact, they went back to work—those of them who still had jobs to take up—at rates prevailing in 1914. Working longer hours for less pay, their union organizations in tatters, mine owners in almost complete control—for miners, the General Strike had proved a humiliating disaster.[37]

Above all, the failure of the General Strike discredited it sufficiently that it would not be resorted to again as a tool in industrial disputes; workers' energies turned toward political, rather than industrial, action. Having been rendered toothless, it seems, unionized workers could now be reconciled to the nation and endowed with the qualities befitting British citizenship. Even before the strike ended,[38] and for many weeks following its defeat, efforts to recuperate the working classes for the nation went on apace. It is from these—largely successful—attempts to recast workers as peace-loving, fair-minded, patriotic and idealistic Englishmen duped into thinking that they acted in the long-standing British tradition of loyalty to their mates that one of the most enduring myths of the General Strike emerged. Once cast as a war against the British nation, an insurrection on the part of an alien group, a soviet-initiated or soviet-inspired revolution, now the General Strike was made out to be an action taken by generous, if misguided, workers on behalf of their less fortunate brothers in the mines. As the *Nation and Atheneum* observed, although the country was "still a long way from peace," the end of the strike had brought about "sheer relief," enabling the "shaping [of] generous phrases about the vindication of Mr Baldwin and the courage of the trade-union leaders, and merging into national self-praise."[39]

In some quarters, it took a day or two before this verdict was reached. The *Daily Mail* initially greeted the end of the strike with strong words against Labour and the trade unions.

It has been called off because it signally failed in the face of the unflinching determination of the British people.... The people who arranged the general strike probably know more about England than they did before they began it. The staunchness of the British nation must have given them a rude shock, and taught them a very much-needed lesson....The T.U.C. itself, which is now hurriedly effacing itself, was a barely disguised Soviet, and, if the spirit of the British nation had not been what it was, might by now have been an actual Soviet ruling a ruined and demoralised people.... The country has come through the deep waters, and it has come through in triumph, setting such an example to the world as has not been seen since the immortal hours of the war. It has fought and defeated the worst form of human tyranny.

But by the next day, the paper had softened its tone, attributing the defeat of the General Strike to "the coolness, and the staunchness, and the patriotism of the entire British people." By the 15th the paper called for generosity to strikers. "The strikers are our own countrymen," it declared, in a dramatic turnaround from just three days prior, "and they have acted under a sense of loyalty to their trade unions. The more generously the employers behave now, the sooner these men will understand how they have been misled." It praised "the rank and file who have, to their credit be it said, generally maintained order and shown an excellent temper," and reminded employers that "there is no spark of vindictiveness in the British character and 'no reprisals' must be the order of the day."[40]

The Times followed the same trajectory, though it took a little more time to change its tone from one of blame to one of reconciliation. It chided those whose

> confused sentimentalism...would have it that neither side has been either defeated or discredited in a fundamental struggle between right and wrong. In a conflict such as that which has been fought out in this country during the last ten days there could be no question of a drawn battle. Its abandonment was one-sided, conclusive, and unconditional.

The paper carried reports of Baldwin's broadcast in which he told the country that "our business is not to triumph over those who have failed in a mistaken attempt. It is rather to rally them together as a whole in an attempt to restore the well-being of the nation;" and published his statement in the Commons that

> the peace that I believe has come—the victory that has been won—is a victory not of any one part of the country, but of the commonsense of the best part of the whole of the United Kingdom, and it is of the utmost importance at a moment like this that the whole British people should not look backwards, but forwards, and that we should resume our work in a spirit of co-operation, putting behind us all malice and all vindictiveness.

But *The Times* could not yet embrace Baldwin's sentiments. The next day, the paper editorialized against the betrayal of the nation by its unionized workforce.

> The men who struck without notice—little though the great majority realized it—had not only broken the law, had not only created

a sense of distrust that threatened to undo the social labours of a whole century, but had also disclaimed that principle of good faith on which all that is most hopeful in every development of the English people is based.

But their willingness to surrender utterly redeemed them sufficiently to enable the country and their employers to reinstate them as members of the nation and as employees. "In abandoning the general strike outright they have at least taken the first step to set themselves right in the eyes of a community which has never yet yielded to threats and has fully proved its capacity to meet them."[41]

Baldwin's efforts at reconciliation better represented public feeling than *The Times'* grudging acceptance of the need to bury the hatchet. Masterson had no fear that workers would be retaliated against. "I do not think that there will be much personal bitterness or victimisation," he stated. "That is not the habit of the English character, especially when it has won. Among most of the employers it is recognised that the rank and file were torn between two loyalties, each, in a sense, disinterested; loyalty to their employers, with whom they had no quarrel, and loyalty to their union, which has been further interpreted, in the terms of a Socialism imported from abroad, as loyalty to their class in a 'class war.' In some of the great newspaper houses the men came out almost in tears, and the managers or proprietors addressed them in terms of conciliation even in the moment of war." Sir John Simon professed to see a new dawn arising from the nightmare of the past nine days. "After a great storm the air is clearing," he cautiously cheered, and urged his constituents and colleagues in a speech in Cleckheaton Town Hall, Yorkshire, on 20 May 1926 to refrain from gloating over the defeat of the strikers. "There is only one victory," he declared,

the victory of the common sense of all classes of the British people . . . . it is not a victory of one party against another, it is just the influence of British character and British temperament finding a way by which we might, acting all together like true comrades, forget the mistakes, retrace the false steps and acknowledge a grievous error.[42]

Before too long, workers who had been castigated as alien revolutionaries and enemies of the British people had become exemplars of the British character. In a letter to *The Times*, C.C. Wakefield applauded "the calmness and good order of the 'non-combatant' men and women who have been so seriously incommoded, and ... the splendid spirit of the police," but he reserved his most fulsome praise for

> the masses of men who have been on strike [who] have also behaved with entirely commendable cheerfulness and self-control. We can truly say that never did a civilised people pass through so serious and potentially disastrous an episode in its history with such cool determination and absence of rancour.... it has been proved that in any great emergency all classes of the nation are prepared to put their country first.

Angus Watson, in a letter to the *Nation and Atheneum*, thrilled to

> the wonderful spirit of altruism that permeates the organized Labour movement. Men in their thousands, I think mistakenly, but none the less sincerely, have risked their whole future in the effort to protect what they conceived to be the best interests of their fellows, and this at great sacrifice to themselves.... We have confirmed the fidelity of our Army, Navy, and Police, all of whom have assisted to preserve our essential services and good order, in some cases at considerable peril to themselves. We have demonstrated again the extraordinary tenacity, determination, and goodwill of the 'man in the street,' who in the face of difficulty and danger has readily stepped in to do what he conceived to be his duty when the nation's rights and liberties were challenged.

The strike had demonstrated, Watson declared, that "the interests of the nation are not divided, but are indivisible."[43]

In a very brief time, "aliens," "enemies," and "revolutionaries" had become the repository of British virtue. Labour leaders had shown "moderation and statesmanship," wrote Simon, they had demonstrated their respect for the law, which "may seem a dusty and insignificant element, but there is an instinct inbred in the British race to submit to it." The strike had put on display the "sanity, the good sense of the British workman." It had demonstrated, said Sir Hall Caine in the *Evening Standard*,

> the splendid spirit of the British people; a spirit such as, in the history of nations, the world has perhaps never known before; first, the splendid spirit of the workers who stood up to the Government in the first instance, by right means or wrong, from no meaner motive than

that of supporting fellow workers whom they believed to be weak and oppressed; and, next, the splendid spirit of the general public who, highly resolved that, come what would, nothing should destroy the stability and welfare of the State.[44]

The strike had become an occasion not to lament or fear but one to celebrate. The *Daily Mail* trumpeted the "World Tributes to Britain. American Joy. Wonderful Sport and Sportsmanship." "John Bull's Dignity. An Example to the World." "In no other country in the world could a domestic conflict of this magnitude and gravity have taken place without bloodshed," crowed Sir John Simon. The Manchester *Guardian* exulted "in the unparalleled pacific character of this great conflict, which has really been the wonder of the world."[45]

Baldwin and Joynson-Hicks were among the few who refused to give up their conviction that trade unions remained potential revolutionary dangers, pawns of Moscow. Baldwin told an audience at Chippenham in June that he wanted "to see our British Labour movement free from alien and foreign heresy," by which he meant an "un-English" "social revolution." "I want to see it pursued and developed on English lines, led by English men." Joynson-Hicks echoed the view that the strike had been instigated by alien forces, though not even he, once the strike was over, could refrain from crediting union leaders with the attributes of true Britishness. In a letter to the Twickenham Conservative Association dated 14 August 1926 he spoke of

how closely the general strike accorded with the plans of Moscow.... while there is no reason to accept at face value the claim of the Communists that they brought about the general strike, it is yet true that such a strike was in their programme, and they and their Soviet masters have not concealed their anger at the return of common sense of the British trade union leaders, and their refusal to allow the strike to develop on revolutionary lines.[46]

This myth about the General Strike overshadowed the virulence of the rhetoric mobilized against workers and Labour politicians and obscured the very real violence that took place in some areas. But the myth-making served to incorporate workers into the body of the nation, allowed them to be recast as fully-fledged Britons possessing all of the sterling qualities of the race. The anxieties and fears they had raised could now be put to rest, and the story of the nation could go on apace with workers playing a big part in it. But if the General Strike appeared to the conservative elements of society to have drawn the teeth of the unions and permitted the integration of workers into the narrative of nation, the potential for the Labour party to act in ways inimical to the interests of the nation, as these conservatives saw it, remained. "The defeat of the strike inclines even the Tory rank and file to mercy towards the Unions," noted the *Nation and Atheneum*. It observed that while "a *détente* has taken place on the part of the Unionist Party" toward the unions, the Labour party had not been cowed. Now that strike activity had been discredited so badly, only politics remained to further working-class aims. "The direct action weapon has been broken," it reminded readers, but "the political weapon is left, and it is sharper than before."[47] Indeed, when the enfranchisement of women between the ages of 21 and 30 appeared to result in the victory of Labour in the 1929 election, the need to eliminate the Labour party from the ranks of "the nation" became even more pressing.

6
Flappers and the Igbo Women's War of 1929 (with Marc Matera)

> To call for troops to deal with an outbreak of women may seem a drastic and unnecessary measure, but these were 'no ordinary women.'[1]
>
> No doubt there are women like ourselves in your country. If need be we will write to them to help us.[2]

Conservatives had attributed their electoral victory of 1924 to the votes of women, whom the party had wooed and the *Daily Mail* targeted in a campaign urging them to cast their ballot for the party that would bring "peace, law and order, and a stable Government." "Women are by nature a conservative force," the *Mail* contended in self-congratulation,

> because they have an innate sense which detects folly and danger by instinct. It is an instinct which serves them better than any verbal logic, and in this case they knew by that instinct that their country's life was threatened. Therefore they flocked in their thousands to the polls, and they voted (as we knew they would) the right way.[3]

This confidence may have led the most surprising of Conservatives, Home Secretary William Joynson-Hicks, to announce almost off-handedly in 1927 the government's intention to bring in a measure to enfranchise women between the ages of 21 and 30.

Feminist organizations and politicians had begun deliberating the question almost immediately after the Representation of the People Act of 1918 gave the vote to women over the age of 30, but serious contemplation of the issue arose only after Joynson-Hicks surprised—and dismayed—a good portion of the party with his statement. At that point, the *Daily Mail* —"perhaps the most powerful newspaper in the

149

kingdom," Joynson-Hicks called it—and, to a much lesser extent, the other major newspapers embarked upon a crusade against the "flapper vote" that reached the point of panic. Two themes dominated the diatribes of the press: the threat of women swamping men and the prospect of the women's vote ushering in an era of socialist and—in the heated rhetoric of the period—bolshevik government. The *Daily Mail*'s Cassandra-like warnings appeared to be borne out when the Labour party was swept into power in the summer of 1929.

Feminism appeared to contemporaries to threaten the social peace.[4] In 1918, women over the age of 30 received the vote, ostensibly in return for their efforts on behalf of the war effort. Some 6 million out of 11 million adult women were enfranchised, the age restriction serving to ensure that women would not enjoy a majority over men, whose numbers had been dramatically reduced by the war. The vote was followed by the Eligibility of Women Act of 1918, which permitted women to stand for parliament. The same year, the bastardy laws of 1872 were amended, thus increasing from five to ten shillings a week the amount a father could be made to pay to support an illegitimate child. In 1919, the passage of the Sex Disqualification Removal Act gave women access to all branches of the legal profession. By 1925, despite the ferocious opposition of entrenched bureaucrats, the civil service admitted women to its competitive examinations, though it refused to pay female civil servants the salaries given to men holding the same position, an inequity that feminists would battle against for years in their equal pay campaign of the 1930s. The Matrimonial Causes Act of 1923, a direct outcome of intense feminist lobbying, eliminated the double standard of divorce. The dissemination of contraceptive information at maternity centers and mothers' clinics, pioneered by birth control advocate Marie Stopes and then established as policy by the Labour government after a long battle among feminists themselves and between men and women within the Labour party, had an immediate impact on family size. In 1913, England and Wales had seen 1,102,500 births. That number dropped to 900,130 births in 1923; 777,520 births in 1926; and to 761,963 births in 1931. The average size of the British family fell from 5.5 in the last quarter of the nineteenth century to 2.2 between 1925 and 1929. In 1928, women finally obtained the franchise on the same terms as it was granted to men.

These were impressive victories by any measure. In addition to welfare benefits implemented during the war to compensate families for the loss of income as men went off to war, some never to return and others to come back too disabled to hold a job—to which, however, married women had no independent right—they improved the lives of many women to a large extent. Certainly these legislative reforms, along with the gains women had made in employment and wages during the war, contributed to an impression that the war had been a boon to women, that it had enhanced their position in the workplace and in political life, and that it had done so at the expense of men.

As early as 1916, in fact, the *Factory Times* urged that "we must get the women back into the home as soon as possible. That they ever left is one of the evil results of the war." Where once women had received accolades of the highest order for their service to the country during war time, by 1918 they were being vilified and excoriated for their efforts. Philip Gibbs returned from the front and charged that ex-soldiers could not find jobs because "the girls were clinging to their jobs, would not let go of the pocket-money which they had spent on frocks." A correspondent for the *Leeds Mercury* wrote in April of 1919 of his "unfeigned pleasure" that women bus conductors and underground drivers would no longer be holding their positions. "Their record of duty well done," he complained, "is seriously blemished by their habitual and aggressive incivility, and a callous disregard for the welfare of passengers. Their shrewish behavior will remain one of the unpleasant memories of the war's vicissitudes." Given the actual nature of the war's vicissitudes, this is quite a profound statement of hostility. As W. Keith pointed out in the *Daily News* in March 1921, in an article titled "Dislike of Women," "the attitude of the public towards women is more full of contempt and bitterness than has been the case since the suffragette outbreaks." The pressures on women to leave their jobs and return to the domestic sphere were intense and often successful. Women did leave their wartime jobs as munitions factories shut down for lack of orders. And beginning in 1921, the traditional employers of women, the great textile factories of Lancashire, began to feel the serious effects of recession, laying off both male and female workers in large numbers, as did other old industries in the north of England like shipbuilding and coal mining. By 1921, fewer women were "gainfully employed," according to the census of that year, than in 1911. Women put out of work by the end of the war and by the beginnings of economic depression refused, as they would not have in the past, to seek employment as domestic servants, an expression of self-regard that certainly helped to drive up their unemployment rates.

But this is only one part of the story. In the south of England, new industries providing household consumer goods by means of large-scale assembly line production began to appear, and they relied upon women to make up the bulk of their semi-skilled workforce. The electrical appliances and the ready-made goods that enabled middle-class women to provide even greater levels of domestic comfort in the interwar years were supplied by wage-earning women. New work opportunities for women in offices as typists, bookkeepers, or cleaning staff, and in shops as assistants and cashiers cropped up, as Britain's economy underwent restructuring from heavy industry in the north to light consumer and service industries in the south.

During this period, women in the Labour party increased their numbers and their influence. A number of women became MPs for Labour— Susan Lawrence, Ellen Wilkinson, and Margaret Bondfield, to name only those who became cabinet ministers—and many, many more served their communities on local governing boards and authorities. To be sure, they faced strongly anti-feminist attitudes within the party, and struggled, usually in vain, to gain acceptance for their demands, but their energies and their activities on behalf of poor and working women helped to improve their lives considerably.

With their enfranchisement in 1918, women joined local branches of the Labour party to a far greater degree than did men. In 1923, 120,000 women belonged to the women's sections of the party; they increased their numbers to as many as 300,000 between 1927 and 1939, comprising at least half of the membership of the party as a whole. In some areas, like Cardiff, they made up as much as three-quarters of the membership. They made their voices heard, urging policies such as the dissemination of contraceptives or family allowances upon their male colleagues. They demanded equal pay for men and women, and, because in only a few jobs could it be claimed that women and men did the same work, comparable pay for women who did work of the same value as men. They strove to endow home- and housework with the dignity of paid labor, and the majority of them believed that married women had the right to work just like their unmarried sisters. In holding this opinion, Labour women departed from the powerful cultural norm that mothers should not work.

The *Daily Mail*'s campaign against the "flapper vote" took place in the context of these dramatic changes in the status of women and in what appeared to many contemporaries to be a decisively negative shift in the relationship between men and women. The boyish young woman against whom the paper railed wore simple, plain-cut, tailored clothing that was best shown off on a lithe, slim, athletic figure with small breasts and narrow hips. She dressed in suits; sported a short haircut, wearing it bobbed, shingled, or Eton-cropped like her elite brothers; she smoked, demonstrated great confidence in herself by her masculine posture and movements, and might boast of a sexual freedom not possible for her prewar sisters. She donned short skirts, drove fast cars, flew airplanes, played golf and tennis with abandon; by her youthful antics, boyish figure, and frantic social pace, she asserted a refusal of maturity and motherhood that elicited adverse comment, especially in the aftermath of a war that had killed half a million men. Her foil, "the modern young man," excited a great deal of negative comment, most of it alluding to his effeminacy and impotence. As early as 1921, the *Daily Mail* worried that "Healthy Young Girls are More Boyish than Boys." In a 1925 front-page story about the disappearance of manliness, the *Daily Express* denounced "The Modern Girl's Brother." In contrast to her—portrayed as strong, healthy, self-confident, and independent—he was described as listless, bored, and dandyish, all "dolled up like a girl and an exquisite without masculinity." *Punch* carried a cartoon in 1928 that depicted a "helpless clinging masculine type" sitting before his assertive, bold fiancé: he with his hands held gracefully in his lap and his legs crossed at the knee, gazing up at her with fawning eyes and sweet expression; she standing above him with her legs astride, hands on hips, in an authoritative manner.[5]

The fear of swamping in the rhetoric mobilized against the "flapper vote" suggested a concern about boundaries, that the lines separating men from women—or, more appropriately, masculine from feminine—had become less distinct and were liable to break down altogether. The anxiety about the blurring of gender lines grew out of the experiences of the Great War, during which the unprecedented opportunities made available to women by the war—their increased visibility in public life, their release from the private world of domesticity, their greater mobility—contrasted sharply with the conditions imposed on men at the front, where they were immobilized and rendered passive in a subterranean world of trenches, emasculated by the horrors they faced and their incapacity to do anything to alter their situation. The anxiety continued in the 1920s, as young women of virtually every class, instead of conforming to a role that assigned to them conventional attributes of self-abnegation, subservience, and motherhood, cut their hair, smoked cigarettes, drove fast cars, wore boyish clothing, danced wildly to a frightening new music associated with American negroes, and comported themselves generally without restraint. "Flappers" conjured up images beyond those of the frivolous, boyish young woman of the jazz age: the term connoted contradictory meanings "of the female as androgyne, a figure characterised as sexless but libidinous; infantile but precocious; self-sufficient but demographically, economically and socially superfluous; an emblem of modern time yet, at the same time, an incarnation of the eternal Eve."[6] Worse still, their numbers, when added to those women voters over the age of 30, surpassed those of men, placing men—and the nation—in a precarious position.

Beginning in 1919 and continuing well into the 1920s, the *Daily Mail* appeared to be obsessed with the numbers of "surplus" women populating Great Britain in the aftermath of the war, on 5 February 1920, for example, expostulating against "A Million Women Too Many" in the "1920 Husband Hunt." It was not merely that these women could never marry; the paper warned that "the social effects of sex disproportion... encourage a lower standard of morality." It decried the "frivolous, scantily clad 'jazzing flapper,' irresponsible and undisciplined," a "large proportion" of whom were "physically attractive girls with strong reproductive instincts and they are ever vying and competing with each other for the scarce and elusive male."[7] This desperate vying for men, explained the *Mail* on 8 August 1921, would follow the evolutionary example of bees: "mankind is going to move towards a state in which there will be a small proportion of mother-women to maintain the race, and a host of male drones," the paper lamented. "They will be supported by the labour of an immense number of sterile female workers. Men will be utterly ousted." As Melman has observed,

> the metaphor of hive bees was immensely emotive, because, if the role of the modern human male was solely to fertilise his mate, then his fate could be compared with that of the drone: annihilation by the race of females he was destined to perpetuate. Implied in the passage is also the notion that sexual intercourse itself is deadly. Similar metaphors of destruction of the male by the new species of women were evoked through the decade. And, in a society living in the shadow of the greatest-ever carnage of males, such metaphors never failed to have an effect.[8]

The conflation of sex and death in the pages of the *Daily Mail* appeared in a variety of venues in the 1920s and 1930s.[9]

In June 1924, the *Daily Mail* heightened its rhetoric, linking the substantial disproportion of women to men to the dangers of extending the electorate by enfranchising women under the age of 30, warning that as the surplus woman "preponderates in numbers she will gradually dominate the electorate."[10] Thus began a campaign against the prospect of enfranchising "flappers" that reached the level of hysteria within a few short years, a campaign that used imagery that linked young women with sexuality, disorder, dominance, profligacy, excess, violence, revolution, threats of emasculation and, finally, the annihilation of men.

Enfranchising women under the age of 30, claimed the *Mail*, risked destabilizing the country. "The constituencies had even now hardly settled down after the disturbances created by the extension of the franchise in 1918, when women first got the vote;" a "leap in the dark" such as that proposed by the government promised to "flood . . . the electoral register with another four or five million voters, mostly irresponsible." This "might lead to a national calamity," the paper cautioned. The "Peril of Feminine Government," the *Mail* warned, was "the most dangerous feature of this proposal;" "the country for all time would be governed by its womenfolk." The 25 April 1927 editorial called the next general election "The Coming Massacre."[11]

Almost from the start, the *Mail* positioned the "flapper vote" alongside the "Bolshevik menace," employing a variety of arguments. One urged that only "Socialists, Communists, Bolsheviks, and Feminist societies" sought this vote, quoting Conservative MP Sir Francis Watson; by forcing Conservatives to attend to an equal franchise bill the government—itself Conservative—would be distracted from fulfilling its campaign promises to ensure "rigid national economy" and protect England "from Zinoviev and his Moscow bandits." Another proclaimed that "Young Women Vote for Reds." Socialists and communists, the paper insisted, enthusiastically supported enlarging the electorate with "irresponsible electors" because they believed that "at least three-fourths of the new votes will be given to them," with which they would win the next election and "enforce mob rule." "Women on the Dole," the *Mail*'s political correspondent claimed, could add "many thousands" of voters to the ranks of the Socialist party, who would lure them to its program "by promises of fuller maintenance by the State." A *Mail* reader wrote in on 8 December 1927 to explain that although she had worked hard to enfranchise women in the past, things had changed and had forced her to reconsider her position. "Bolshevism was not the menace that it is to-day," she stated, and as most of the newly enfranchised would vote Labour, she could not support an act that would enable trade unions to exercise undue power. In perhaps the baldest expression of flappers as communists, the *Mail* on 31 August 1928 carried a headline that read "New Moscow Order to Our Reds . . . . Attempt to Capture Flapper Vote." The story itself contained no reference to the purported instruction.[12]

The *Mail* promised that the flapper vote would contribute to violence and disorder throughout the nation and the empire. The vast majority of them would vote socialist, it claimed, and socialism would produce "tyranny and violence." "The backbone in Ireland of Mr. de Valera's party of violence and revolution is the young woman voter," declared the editorial of 23 November 1927. A 30 July 1928 headline reporting on "Communist Women's London Trip" sat just above another declaring "Moscow's War Plans in India." The vote was "like putting a sharp knife in the hands of a child," wrote one reader of the *Mail* on 14 December 1927. To another, giving young women the vote would be "giving over the country completely to feminism—a far more sinister enemy than any foreign power." The country was "approaching the abyss," wrote the *Mail* on 20 December 1927.[13]

One reader of the *Mail* wrote to the paper on 6 December 1927 to warn against enfranchising the "irresponsible women who now wantonly defy the law that no woman may behave indecently. Daily millions of women defy the law and walk about half naked in the public streets." In a feature entitled "The Future of Women," Michael Harlen asked whether women would oust men from business or politics. "What will they wear?" he continued. "They can't wear less. Or can't they?" he wondered. As if in response, the *Mail* carried an editorial about the possibility of women displaying their "Bare Legs" at Wimbledon in the same space as its editorial on the results of the general election. Two days later, it carried a news story entitled "Stockings or No Stockings, To-day's problem for Wimbledon" under the banner "Socialist Prime Minister in Power To-Day."[14]

The *Daily Express* focused its attention less on the numbers of women who would vote under the new bill and more on how they would use their votes, warning readers against the "petticoat government" that would ensue because the cabinet had taken "the Plunge." Its 14 April 1927 front page carried a column headlined "Russian Forces Massing," next to which sat a cartoon of a modern woman with a short skirt and bare legs posed nonchalantly with cigarette in hand, entitled "The New Dictator," next to which stood a column titled "Women's Bill Next Session." The editorial that day, subtitled "Votes for 'Flappers,'" cautioned that "the opening of this vast door will mean a complete re-orientation of our politics." The 15 April 1927 edition of the *Express* positioned two unrelated stories under a picture of three working-class women titled "What Our New Dictators are Saying." The one, "Man Killed in a London Bank," stood immediately next to the other entitled "Votes for Women at Twenty-One." A 25 April 1927 cartoon headed

"Independence" depicted a flapper with bobbed hair and cigarette, the caption below reading, "The modern girl knows her own mind, does not seek advice or tolerate control, and she will certainly vote without taking counsel from anybody." The editorial that day carried a heated attack on "a persistent group of spinsters" seeking to persuade the Labour party to place the dissemination of information about birth control by the Ministry of Health on its official program. "If these women have their way," the editorial warned, "the parliamentary Opposition—which may possibly again supply the Government of this country—is to be driven into accepting a policy of race suicide, and a state department is to be used for the gradual destruction of the nation which it is supposed to serve and preserve." The "racial threat" posed by birth control, the impetus to "promiscuity" it entailed, charged the editorial board, would "destroy the basis of marriage," "abolish the family," "annihilate the system on which the nation is based," and "turn the country into a chattering monkeyhouse."[15]

The bill to enfranchise women between the ages of 21 and 30 encountered little realistic opposition in the House of Commons—the second reading passed by a vote of 387–10—though it generated some heated rhetoric from a segment of the Conservative party, "protesting with vehemence and even with rage against" Joynson-Hicks' remarks in favor of the bill, as one bitter opponent put it. Joynson-Hicks characterized the deep anger about the bill as a "kind of undercurrent . . . in conservative circles of hostility towards the Prime Minister and his Government." He opened the second reading with the observation that the equal franchise bill would broaden the base on which democracy rested, providing greater stability for the freedoms and liberties enjoyed by Britons. He challenged any member of the House who would "suggest that he fears the people, . . . who fears the consequences of the democratic vote" to take heart from the lessons of history and embrace the greater representation of the people. Conceding that the current majority of three million male voters over female voters would be replaced by a two million majority of women over men, he dismissed the concern of opponents "that the control of political power will be transferred from men to women," daring them to

> say that women are unfit intellectually for the vote, that their judgment is not as sound as that of men, that with the progress of women in all stages of society, in all businesses and in all professions, what has been so startling in its rapidity, they are to be exempted from one

right, and one right only, in this country, that of exercising their vote for a Member of Parliament.[16]

One MP, Lieutenant-Colonel Sir F. Hall of Dulwich, did aver that his opposition to the bill stemmed from his long-held conviction that "the country should be represented in this House by the male sex," but the other MPs who voted against the bill framed their arguments more circumspectly. They did not oppose women's rights to equality, they declared, they opposed a measure that would place women in a majority over men at the polls. Designed as an act of justice to young women, it would, more accurately, asserted Brigadier-General George Cockerill, "inflict a far graver injustice on men, taken as a whole." "Women will have absolute supremacy at the polls," he warned. "Now women will have both the will and the way." Questioning "whether women ought to be the determining factor in our political life," Cockerill offered up his answer: "if either sex is to be supreme at the polls," he stated bluntly, "I would prefer to see, quite frankly, men put in the supremacy. Outside this House I do not believe there are very many people who want to see men put in a permanent minority in every constituency in the country." In response to a colleague's interjection that they should be "Masters in their own house," Cockerill added, "Not subordinate to the mistresses in their own house." He urged that the bill be altered to ensure that parity of male and female voters be achieved; in an aside remarkable for what it revealed about the depth of his anxieties, Cockerill observed that one way of dealing with the unfortunate fact that more girls grew to adulthood than men, despite the preponderance of male over female births, was "to murder the women innocents," an option, he hastened to say, he did not advocate. "I do not think we have any right to abdicate the scepter of political power," he intoned, "and, as for women, I think it would become woman better to assume the robe of Portia and deal out evenhanded justice between the sexes, rather than to wear the garment of Shylock and clutch at the jeweled orb of power."[17]

Samuel Samuel announced four times in his speech that "women are not unfit to vote." He reminded the House, however, that "we are not dealing with parochial questions," presumably the ones he meant when he said that "they are perfectly capable of forming an opinion as to their own requirements."

We have to deal with great questions of Empire, and with international questions. If we were dealing with the question of a new handle for the parish pump, I quite agree that we should get very good advice and assistance from a larger electorate.... We are going by the Measure to give to people who know absolutely nothing beyond the parish pump—for, after all, how many of these new electors realize the immensity of the British Empire or of British interests outside our Empire?—we are going to give to them the enormous power of regulating the foreign and Colonial policy of this country.

Sir C. Oman echoed Samuel's disquiet, adding a frightening allusion to the scenario by recalling the last time he had voted against his party's leadership in the matter of the Government of India bill. "On the heads" of those Conservatives who, as now, had voted with their party against their principles "are all the blood and turmoil and trouble that have come in India as a result of that Bill. Let every man take warning from that to-night," he declared, comparing the violence of colonial revolt with what would certainly arise were women to gain a preponderance of political power.[18]

Major G.M. Kindersley's objection to the bill derived from the "vast, fundamental and permanent constitutional change" that would result from giving women not equality with men but "permanent political supremacy" over them. Such an action, coming at a time when no effective second chamber ("the Second Chamber is emasculated," he observed, in referring to the all-male House of Lords in telling imagery) served to counterbalance women's majority, meant that "the political supremacy which you are giving to women is absolute." "The woman's view shall prevail," he warned. And then he raised the specter that had long been at the heart of the opposition to women's suffrage—the prospect of sex war. This line of reasoning rested upon the "physical force" argument that had dogged suffragists for some 60 years: that the "ultimate sanction which rests behind all law," as Kindersley put it, is force. "Supposing by the votes of women legislation was passed in this country which men deeply resent," he hypothesized. "How is that legislation going to be enforced?" This scenario, he warned, however remote, was a possibility, and it "would bring about sex war—inevitably it would bring about sex war."[19]

As I have argued elsewhere, conjuring the possibility of sex war had long been a staple of anti-suffrage strategy, and the threat of it by means of conflating sex war with the real war being waged in Europe was used, paradoxically, in 1917, to justify allowing women to vote.[20] Certainly the war informed the thinking of politicians as they wrangled over the extension of the franchise to younger women. In summing up the government's position, Baldwin instanced the experience of the war on several occasions. To his mind, and that of many, many others, women had earned the vote in the first place through their contributions to the war effort; it is clear that that particular rationale—and the unspoken but ever-present anxieties it provoked—continued to resonate in 1928 as the elusive return to normalcy still loomed large. Baldwin portrayed the granting of equal franchise as "the final stage in the union of men and women working together for the regeneration of their country and for the regeneration of the world."[21]

Cockerill and the rest of the opposition continually referred to the overwhelming superiority of numbers women would enjoy should the bill become law. The fear that men would be "swamped" by women appeared in the rhetoric of virtually every member who spoke against the bill. "The men's vote will be swamped," warned Cockerill. "We shall have a majority of 2,200,000 women over men," noted Applin. Harmsworth—Lord Rothermere of the *Daily Mail*—decried "these continual dilutions of the electorate" by women's suffrage bills that had helped to produce "mobs of voters," "vast mobs of people who have the vote." The 1918 reform act had limited voting to women over 30 precisely because "the men who were coming back from the Front would have their votes swamped by the great number of new voters who would be put on the register. Might I ask what has changed that reason?"[22]

Adrian Bingham argues convincingly that the *Daily Mail*'s obsession with the "flapper vote," which exceeded all bounds of proportion, was actually an obsession with socialism. Its owner, Lord Rothermere, feared that women under 30 would flock to the Labour party, bringing in a government that, he believed, would destroy the country. Certainly we should accept at face value the conviction that bolshevism constituted a danger to Britain; but there is more at work here. The *Mail* also utilized the concept of the "feminine" to represent the dangers of bolshevism, and that usage should alert us to something deeper going on. "Flappers" called forth ideas of frivolity, irresponsibility, and a set of sexual behaviors that constituted a significant break with the mores and morals of the past. But they could also represent instability of a more profound, more threatening sort, a transgression of boundaries that could signal the annihilation of the self. The subject of the interwar period experienced himself—and this claim should be extended to include women as well—as "shattered." The subjects whose formative identities derived from the experiences of the war felt a desperate need to protect themselves against the chaotic forces that threatened fragmentation and dissolution. Two of Rothermere's sons died in the Great War, a loss that left him "shattered," as one relative described him. His embrace of

Mussolini and Hitler as exemplars of strong government is not merely indicative of his desire for a British equivalent, in which capacity, he believed for a time, Oswald Mosley could serve. Bingham shows that Rothermere's flirtation with fascism was not a short-lived, misguided display of sentiment; his admiration for the policies of Hitler and Mussolini continued long after his split with Mosley in 1934. I would argue that Rothermere's infatuation with strong, masculine leaders was not simply "a means of remedying what he perceived to be a loss of the virility and active patriotism that had previously marked the British Empire and its leaders," as Bingham puts it. It also constituted a yearning for a figure possessing the power to keep the threat of annihilation at bay.[23]

While the *Times* and the *Guardian* did not participate in anything like the *Mail's* campaign against the "flapper" vote, and explicitly distanced themselves from the use of what they saw as a derogatory term, their coverage of the debate over the bill and of the election of 1929 echoed many of the *Mail's* charges, if obliquely or in more moderate language. In some instances, reporters raised charges like those that claimed the new voters were "flighty, uneducated, irresponsible young things," or that "the fate of the country is now being handed over to its most irresponsible citizens" in order to dismiss them, and then used the term "flapper" to describe new voters in a different article. In other instances, the juxtaposition of articles about the women's vote against those about the General Strike of 1926, disorder caused by communists or socialists in Berlin or Paris, or calls by readers or politicians for "a stable government" linked women to the very incidents of disorder, danger, and bolshevism that the *Mail* railed against.[24]

More directly, both the *Guardian* and the *Times* declared that they did not know what could be expected of these new voters. They were "inscrutable" and "puzzling," an "enigma," a "riddle," the "incalculable element" in the election. The purported unknowability of women contributed to the derision with which the flapper was met—she was fickle—the "Girl Who Changed Her Mind," as the *Guardian* portrayed one of them the day after the poll; she was frivolous—"I am voting for Mr. Churchill's party because his dog belongs to the Wagtails' Club, and my dog is a member too;" she was ignorant—"I thought Lloyd George was a Conservative." Even MacDonald, whose Labour party, it was supposed correctly, stood to gain the most from the influx of new voters, could muster only a conditional vote of confidence in the women he hoped would sweep him into office. "She has brought a serious mind to her responsibilities," he noted of the new voter, "which has the promise that on Thursday she will deliver a sane judgment," leaving open the possibility that she might not.[25]

Above all, the *Times* and the *Guardian*, as well as the *Mail* and the *Express* and the MPs who voted both for and against the equal franchise bill, obsessed about the numbers of women voters who would be enfranchised and the size of the majority they would hold over men. Even as the papers editorialized that fears about the existence of a woman's bloc were unfounded, as the *Guardian* did on 20 May 1929, their coverage belied any such sanguine notions. In contrast to that of the *Mail*, coverage of the debate over the bill by the *Times* and the *Guardian* was muted; the papers reported the debates but said little else. Once the voting register was thrown open on 1 May 1929, however, both papers trained eyes on the numbers: from 1 May to 1 June, they published column after column of numbers, totting up the men's and women's votes like debits and credits on a balance sheet. "Big Preponderance of Women," proclaimed the *Times*; "Woman's Dominance," echoed the *Guardian*, listing those constituencies "Where Men Are Outnumbered Greatly." "Men Outnumbered by Women," the *Times* intoned the next day, while the *Guardian* purported to have discovered a few "Men's Strongholds." In a few constituencies, "the men are swamped," it noted. On 10 May 1929, it was able to report "A Good Day for the Men," finding that men were "Holding Their Own" in a few boroughs and counties. May 15 found "The Women's Lead" in Scotland and London; by 18 May, when all the figures were in, women voters held a "Lead of 1,3000,000." The *Times* announced on 20 May that the new electorate included "Seven Million New Voters;" five million of those were women. "Women voters are considerably in excess of men," in most of the divisions, noted the *Guardian*, and "could turn the election."[26]

They did. The fears of people like Rothermere came to pass, as it became clear in the days immediately following the election that the new women voters had gone disproportionately for the Labour party, giving it the largest share of seats in the House of Commons, though not an outright majority. The *Times* informed its readers of "Labour Gains" on 31 May, noting that "in some of the polling stations ... the male voters were in a hopeless minority." The Labour party's "Gains and Losses" appeared in a column immediately next to one reporting that the king had suffered "A Feverish Attack" and was "Confined to Bed at Windsor." One presumes it was not the election results that had made him ill, but readers might be excused for having thought so. "The New Voters for Labour," those who gave "The Lion's Share" of their ballots to Ramsay MacDonald's party, had, the *Guardian* implied through the positioning of its articles, brought into office "A Militant I.L.P. Group." In celebration of their victory, the paper continued in the next column, "Great Crowd Invades King's Cross," where "Mr. MacDonald Mobbed," "Swept Off His Feet."[27]

The numbers demonstrated that women would "swamp" men. "Sweeping Majorities for Women Voters" existed in virtually every constituency, the *Mail* declared. Though more subtle than the *Mail* or the *Express*, the *Times* and the *Guardian* shared in those papers' fears of a great tidal wave of women overcoming men, a theme that marked coverage of the equal franchise bill from the start. Concerns that men's votes would be "diluted" cropped up occasionally; most often, the papers expressed anxieties about sweeping away the boundaries that separated men from women and self from other. The equal franchise bill would cause "the opening of the floodgates to flappers," insisted L.J. Maxse, the editor of the *National Review*. "Women's 'Equal Rights' Storm," announced the *Mail* on 29 August 1928, reporting on the meeting of "Feminists of All the World" in France. Accounts of "How Men Will Be Swamped" appeared regularly, as did letters objecting to the "swamping" of the electorate by female voters. The Labour victory prompted the *Mail* to bemoan the "rising tide" of socialism that required great effort on the part of Conservatives if their seats in all constituencies were not to be "swept away." Theirs had been a "shattering defeat," the paper declared, and necessitated the elimination of the "She-Men" who had brought it upon the party by extending the franchise to women, the very appellation speaking volumes about the blurring of gender boundaries that so occupied the unconscious thoughts of so many interwar Britons. As one historian suggests, it cannot be mere coincidence that "the year of the 'flapper' vote saw the publication of *Death of a Hero*, a fiercely misogynistic work in which liberated women betray their soldier menfolk." The conviction that women had been responsible for the line against bolshevism being breached rendered them dangerous, capable of the most extreme betrayal.[28]

In a dramatic coincidence, one of the first crises the Labour party faced brought to the surface precisely the conflation of women with sexuality and violence and the swamping of boundaries that had exercised conservatives throughout the campaign to enfranchise women under 30. In November and December of 1929, a remarkable series of demonstrations, protests, risings, and riots involving tens of thousands of women took place in southeast Nigeria. The Aba Riots, as the British dubbed them at the time in what one supposes was a bid to efface their extraordinary nature, are known to their participants and subsequent African memory and historiography as the *Ògù Umùnwaàyi*, the Igbo Women's War. In the course of it, more than 50 Igbo women were killed by British troops.[29]

The war broke out on 24 November 1929, when rumors that the British planned to tax women reached the village of Oloko in southeast Nigeria. In response to what appeared to be efforts to assess their wealth by the warrant chief, Okugo, a large number of Igbo women surrounded his compound and "sat on" him, a customary practice when men committed offenses against women. When "sitting on a man," women danced and sang until the object of their grievance acknowledged his offense and promised to make restitution.[30] In this particular instance, Okugo not only refused to admit to any wrong-doing on his part, he set the members of his compound on the women, causing injury to eight of them. Angered by their treatment, the women sent a deputation to the District Officer at Bende, Captain Cook, to complain about Okugo's actions.

While the deputation of Oloko women conferred with Cook, women from Aba, Owerri, and Ikot Ekpene arrived in Oloko, and, upon hearing that Cook had agreed to try Okugo, moved on to Bende, gathering up other women en route. By the time they arrived, their numbers had reached into the thousands, and Cook had handed over his commission to Captain Hill. "The women," Hill testified later, "numbering over ten thousand, were shouting and yelling round the office in a frenzy. They demanded [Okugo's] cap of office, which I threw to them and it met the same fate as a fox's carcass thrown to a pack of hounds." Satisfied by Hill's promise that Okugo would be tried for assault and that women would not be taxed, the women disassembled and returned to their villages without incident.[31]

Persistent rumors of taxation of women and news of the women's victory at Bende spread to other towns and villages, where women met in late November and early December to discuss their situation. On 9 December, a crowd of women estimated to number 1000 attacked the Native Court at Owerrinta, knocking the caps from the heads of warrant chiefs, damaging property, and destroying documents. The next day, 10 December, crowds of women gathered at Aba, where they again attacked the Native Court and then looted Barclay's Bank and a number of European warehouses, where palm oil, the staple product of women's economic activity, was stored. A week later, on 16 December, at Utu Etim Ekpo, in Calabar Province, women attacked the Native Court, a warehouse, and the houses of the clerks employed there. When they turned their attention to demanding a meeting with the District Officer, troops were called in; when the women insisted upon proceeding to the District Officer's offices, the troops opened fire on them with rifles and a Lewis gun, killing 18.

The following day, 17 December 1929, a bigger crowd of women met at Opobo, where they demanded a written statement from the District Officer that asserted, among other things, that women would not be taxed. While they waited for the agreement to be typed up, the women grew increasingly restless, pushing on the fence that held them outside the yard of the District Office and offering up insults to the troops inside the fence line. Just as the fence began to give way, the lieutenant in charge of the troops gave an order to fire. The soldiers shot and killed 32 women; an additional eight women were pushed by the retreating crowd into the river below and drowned; 31 women lay wounded by gunfire. As Lt. Col. P. F. Pritchard explained in his short narrative of his experiences during the women's war, entitled "More Deadly Than the Male,"

> To call for troops to deal with an outbreak of women may seem a drastic and unnecessary measure, but these were "no ordinary women." In toughness and a potential ability to make trouble they were a far more potent force than their menfolk. Seventy years before this date, an army from the neighboring territory of Dahomey had invaded Nigeria and attacked Abeokuta. One third of this invasion force were women and the fame of the "Amazons" of Dahomey became legendary.[32]

Historians have pointed out that African women constituted for British males the quintessential "other," a tantalizing and terrifying mélange of "she-devil" and "sexual temptress." The language by means of which British military and police officers, colonial agents in Nigeria, colonial and political officials in London, and other observers described and tried to explain the events and behaviors of the Igbo women betray a sensibility, a subjectivity, that could not easily withstand what appeared to be assaults, even the unconscious threat of psychic annihilation, posed by the women. The British described the events of the Igbo Women's War in language redolent with sexual panic and even hysteria, in imagery consistent with the threats of fragmentation and dissolution that characterized much interwar representation of the self.[33]

Sexual undertones and the conflation of sex and death in the minds of the British authorities in Nigeria appear regularly in their accounts of the women's war. From even the most reticent testimony the unease and discomfort provoked by the sexual aspects of the women's behavior becomes readily apparent. "Sitting on a man," for instance, the event that initiated the women's war, involved women dancing and singing their grievances, and literally placing their bodies upon the offending party. We do not know exactly what the women sang as they "sat on" the various local chiefs or danced in protest against colonial authority, but some hints emerge from various sources from which we can piece together a plausible case that the songs were of a nature to cause British men and women to blush. Margaret Green, a trained anthropologist who undertook studies of Igbo women in the immediate aftermath of the women's war, recounted the lyrics of the songs the women sang as they danced and "sat on" miscreants in a particular village. "I am seeking someone to have sexual connection with me," went the chorus of one song. "Women who will not come out into this place, let millipede go into her sex organs, let earthworm go into her sex organs," ran another designed to "induce women... to turn out in force." Another song contained lyrics about "sex organs being bright... during connection.... sex organ is good to hold in hand like flute. Only there is no place one is holding it with hand." Green described in imagery recalling the mythic, monstrous, fantastic visions of "fierce Amazons" in the "matriarchies of West Africa" a "sitting on" ritual she witnessed.

> I saw a woman dart across the yard to join the dancers in a succession of wild leaps, her arms outstretched and the long, hanging breasts that so many of these women have adding to the grotesque effect.... there was a menace in their dancing that must have been highly unpleasant for the object of it. They pranced aggressively, sometimes holding their buttocks with their hands, sometimes sticking them out and shaking them; or they advanced making sexually suggestive gestures, and the quality of their laughter again conveyed their feeling of obscenity.

She described this night of ritual "sitting on" an "orgy."[34]

Later sources suggest what might have been sung and done to men. T. Obinkaram Echewa's fictional account of the women's war, *I Saw the Sky Catch Fire*, published in 1992, includes a scene in which the protagonist's grandmother participates in a singing and dancing action against a man who has beaten his wife. "Ozurumba, Ozurumba," the women chanted, "you like to beat your wife! /You will beat all of us tonight,/Until your arms fall off!/Ozurumba, Ozurumba, you have the biggest prick in town/You will fuck all of us tonight,/Until your prick falls off!" When Ozurumba tried to flee, the women

> jerked off his loincloth so that he was completely naked. A roar of laughter and applause arose from the women as the strip of loincloth passed as trophy among the women.... The women pushed Ozurumba to the ground and spread him out, face up, holding his hands and legs so he could not struggle free. Then they took turns sitting on him, pulling up their cloths and kirtles to their bare buttocks and planting their nakedness on every exposed element of his body.[35]

Although we cannot absolutely assert that Echewa's novelistic depictions or Green's ethnographic depictions accurately reflect the nature of the events witnessed by or told to the British in 1929 and 1930, British and native officials describing the women's actions invoked the same, if less graphic, images of sexual behavior to explain what had gone on and why they reacted the way they did. In testimony before a commission of inquiry investigating the "Aba riots," a native interpreter declined to articulate for the justices what one of the women involved had just told members, explaining that her words were not ones that could properly be stated before the court. British officers were less hesitant to offend the commission's sensibilities. Lt. Col. Pritchard told the commission that the women at Utu Etim Ekpo with whom he came into contact were led by

> an old woman who had no clothes on, except some leaves round her neck. The women seemed to be under the influence of this woman, and they were acting in a strange manner. Some lay on the ground and kicked their legs into the air, some passed most offensive remarks and made obscene gestures.

The Medical Officer at Opobo, Edward James Crawford, testified that the women who protested there had come from the town of Doctor's Farm–"the women there are mostly prostitutes, there must be hundreds of them," he claimed–and that they had arrived at Opobo "stripped" of their clothing. "I have been five years in this country," he went on, "and I have never seen such a truculent crowd before in this country. The women normally wear a great deal of clothing and nearly all wear jumpers and none of them carry sticks. This morning the majority were stripped to the waist." A commission report, accepting uncritically Crawford's unsubstantiated and false claim that the "women of loose character" from Doctor's Farm attacked and looted the warehouses of Messrs. G.B. Ollivant & Co., then made its own conflation of sexually immoral women and assault and asserted, wrongly, that the women at Opobo demanded, in addition to the abolition of taxation, that prostitutes not be arrested. "The solicitude [for prostitutes] thus shown throws a light upon the class of women of which the ringleaders were composed," its authors stated. In yet another collapse of sex and violence, the commission reported that

> the greater part, if not all, of the women were armed with stout cudgels and in place of the voluminous clothing usually worn by the native women in Opobo, were for the most part stripped to the waist and wore only loin cloths.... It was therefore manifest that their intentions were hostile and that their attitude was far removed from that of women who were going to have a peaceful meeting with the District Officer.

These sexually threatening women promised to overwhelm the officers and troops within the fenced-in area; when the fence gave way the troops fired on the crowd of women. Though British authorities later declared that the women had been charging the troops when they were shot, the inquest reports show that most of the wounds were inflicted on the sides or the backs of the women's heads and bodies, indicating that they were in fact running away from the gunfire when they were hit.

British officers involved in the shootings repeatedly equated women's sexuality with the threat of dissolution, with the loss of boundaries and even death. Lt. Richard Hill described the crowd of women

> pressing against the light bamboo fence, they were all shouting and waving sticks. I estimated the crowd at 400 women of all ages; there were no children; some were nearly naked wearing only wreaths of grass round their heads, waist and knees and some were wearing tails made of grass.... Some abused me in English and one took off her loin cloth and told me that I was the son of a pig and not of a woman. I was told that the others were speaking in native dialect were telling the soldiers to cut their throats.... Each time a new batch of women arrived the frenzy of the mob increased.[36]

Because "there were no children," and "some were nearly naked," Hill believed, violence at the hands of these women must almost inevitably follow. Indeed, British colonial officials discussed the presence of naked

African women and the threat of destruction at their hands as if they were indistinguishable; the women's nakedness ensured "that their intentions were hostile." The senior British official at Consular Beach, District Officer Whitman, repeatedly interpreted nudity as malicious or violent intent in his representations of the women. "A large crowd of women was met," Whitman stated in his report on the incident, "dressed in narrow loin-cloth, not in their customary, clothes worn on peaceful occasions . . . . very soon a continuous stream of excited, gesticulating women began to enter the station and make towards the District Office."[37] The coroner for Opobo stated in the report from his initial inquiry into the shooting, "if they came to the station merely to put their grievances before the D.O. they would have been dressed in their ordinary clothes and would never have come armed."[38]

For British colonial officials, the preconceived image of the African female body as simultaneously saturated with sexual desire and a source of destruction rendered the tension all the more acute, illustrated in the accounts of these men by their associations of women's uncovered bodies with their "threatening" or "menacing" demeanor. The "disorder" experienced by the men mirrored their own internal sense of self, provoking such acute anxiety over the loss of their own boundaries as individuated subjects that it seemed that the only possible release from the tension was violent aggression, the rejection and even destruction of the perceived threat: they believed they had no choice but to fire on the women. As Captain James explained,

> the mobs at Utu Etim Ekpo had no fear of the troops and were making a deliberate attack with the object of swamping the troops and so disarming and destroying them. The situation was one of extreme danger to the country, as any success would in my opinion have led to a universal and frenzied rising in the District.[39]

The notion of taking the offensive before the women could "swamp" them recurs in the representations of the British soldiers and officials, constituting their explanation for the shootings at Opobo and Utu Etim Ekpo during the women's war. As one officer asserted in a revealing remark during the coroner's initial inquiry, "my platoon of 26 men was in danger of being swamped by an overwhelming mass if action was not taken at once." When asked by a member of the commission, "what were the women doing? Were they merely demonstrating, or were they out for mischief?" he said, "I am definitely certain they were out for mischief. I have seen mobs in Ireland and India, and these were certainly more riotous than any I have ever seen before. They came towards me and nothing could have stopped them." This officer experienced the crowd of African women demonstrators as extreme chaos as well as the ultimate threat to the "proper" order. In light of this unprecedented threat, it seemed obvious to Browning that when "they came towards" him he had no choice but to shoot.[40] He and others felt they could not risk physical contact with the crowd of women: it would effect their annihilation.

The women's war commands a central place in African history and ethnography; its drama, impact, and significance for Nigerian colonial and national developments have ensured that virtually any scholar of Africa, no matter the field, knows about it. This is not the case for those who study Britain. The women's war does not appear in British textbooks or monographs about the period; British historians, with one apparent exception,[41] know nothing about it, a lapse that mirrors the lack of attention given the war by the British press, the British parliament, and British public opinion. The women's war, contrary to the expectations of the most senior members of the Colonial Office, not only evoked no outrage whatsoever, it caused hardly a ripple on the pages of the *Times,* the *Guardian,* the *Daily Mail,* the *Daily News,* or in parliamentary debates and proceedings. In the scant coverage that did appear for brief moments, it would have been possible to hear of the women's actions and not understand that they had been undertaken by women at all.

Granted, the women's war did not confront the British public with the slaughter of 400-odd unarmed men, women, and children who had been gathered at Amritsar in 1919. But the loss of life of 58 women should have sparked some outrage among the British public. Colonial officials certainly thought that it would, asserting in private correspondence that, as Governor Graeme Thomson telegraphed to Secretary of State Lord Passfield (Sidney Webb), "I considered that an immediate enquiry into this matter was essential in order to satisfy public opinion both here and in England." Under-Secretary of State Drummond Shiels wrote a memo marked "Very Urgent" to his superiors about the "Nigerian Shootings," warning that the

> feeling in the House and in the country will be greatly aroused over the happenings in Nigeria.... the story does not read well and there is certain to be a strong feeling expressed that certain people have blundered, and that they are being screened by superiors. I do not say that this is true, but we shall have great difficulty in the House

in explaining the killing of 35 [handwritten insert] women by rifle fire and the drowning of 8 by being pushed into the river by what was apparently a panic stricken mob.... It is a black chapter in our West African history and will be described as another Amritsar with the worst aspect that all but one of the 36 victims [number 44 has been struck through in the typescript] were women:[42]

The Times first carried the story on 13 December 1929, under the headline, "Native Unrest in Nigeria. Europeans Assaulted." The entire article read:

> Much unrest has developed in some parts of South-Eastern Nigeria. Trouble broke out in a village about 15 miles distant from Opobo, where a political officer was attacked, a native Court burnt down, and telegraphic communications were temporarily destroyed. A large force of police is now in the area.
>
> Minor troubles in the nature of demonstrations have occurred at Umuahia and other places in the neighbourhood. On Tuesday demonstrations by several hundreds of native women took place in Aba itself, and they were repeated yesterday. Europeans were assaulted, the offices of Barclays Bank were rushed, two European stores were forced and partially looted, and the District Officer's headquarters were attacked. Reinforcements of police were obtained and a small detachment of troops arrived this morning. The situation is well in hand.[43]

The fact that women demonstrated is mentioned in paragraph two of the story, but it comes relatively late, and appears to have been obscured by the information given in the first paragraph, by the use of the term "minor" to describe the demonstrations, and by the emphasis placed on the assault on Europeans, which, in fact, did not take place. When next *The Times* reported on the events, on 16 December, no mention of women was made at all. A 19 December story referred to "clashes with natives" having taken place in Opobo without designating that those natives were women, although in the section on "Parliament" in the same edition, the paper reproduced the statement of Shiels, in reply to questions raised by two MPs. Shiels noted that all of the casualties at Opobo had been women, but it would have been hard to discern from his speech that the "rioters" were exclusively female. The *Daily Mail*, by contrast, headed its short report that day with "18 Women

Shot," telling readers that "a large crowd proceeded to loot and destroy property," compelling the police to fire. "It is not yet known how many of the 18 women hit were killed or have died from injuries." The following day, *The Times* carried another story on "The Unrest in S.E. Nigeria" in which its correspondent noted that the station at Opobo "was crowded with women," but other sections of the text imply that it was, at the very least, a mixed crowd, and that men, not women, played the key role in the rioting.[44] The *Mail* reported on that same incident on 20 December 1929, failing to note that the "rioters" and "disorderly crowds" were comprised almost exclusively of women. A four-sentence story in the 21 December issue of *The Times* reporting that the crisis seemed to have passed made no mention of women, but on 24 December, Christmas Eve, readers of the paper learned more about the nature of the riots. Under the headline, "The Unrest in S.E. Nigeria. Casualties Among Native Women," they learned that

> in the early morning of December the District Officer met a large mob of women armed with sticks and parleyed with them for hours. War canoes arrived to carry off loot from the factories and men armed with machetes landed and hung around the outskirts of the mob. A rush of the mob cut off the District Officer and a small party of 12 police from the rest of the town, leaving Europeans defenceless. Fortunately, at 8 o'clock in the morning one platoon of troops under Lieutenant R.M. Hill, The Welch Regiment and Nigeria Regiment, arrived and forced its way through the mob to join the District Officer. Parley with the mob continued, and Lieutenant Hill was hit with sticks. The mob gradually pushed back the District Officer and Lieutenant Hill until the troops had their backs to the office wall. Lieutenant Hill warned the mob more than 10 times that he would be compelled to fire unless disorder ceased, and fired his revolver as a warning.

> At last, as attempts were being made to snatch rifles from the troops and the District Officer was being attacked, Lieutenant Hill gave orders to fire. The rush of the mob pushed some women into the river, and eight of them drowned. Nineteen women and one man were killed by the rifle fire and 10 women died of wounds. The officers on the spot are satisfied that to open fire was the only possible course to save life and property.... The only other casualties are reported from Abako, where a frenzied mob attacked the station on December 11 and the police were compelled to fire, six women being killed.

Here, too, although it should have been clearer to the reading public that the rioters were women, it was possible to believe that they had been instigated and led by men. Coverage on 29 December referred to an attack on a native chief by "neighbours" that resulted in the deaths of four people and the wounding of 20 more. Only at the end of the short article, when the paper noted that "the general position of the disturbed areas has improved, and the women are returning to their villages," would readers have learned that the "neighbours" who assaulted the native chief were women. The *Mail's* story was virtually identical.[45]

Articles pertaining to the "disturbances" in *The Times* on 30 December 1929, 31 December 1929, 8 January 1930, and 30 January 1930 failed to identify the "rioters" and "looters" as women. Finally, on 31 January, the paper reported on the establishment of a commission of inquiry into the "unrest" in southeast Nigeria and in the last paragraph noted that

a feature of the disturbances was that women were the actual aggressors and were put forward, it is stated, in the belief that the authorities would not fire on them. This supposition proved incorrect. At Opobo, the British officer, after parleying with the women for hours without effect and finding that they had driven the troops to the wall of the station and were in the act of snatching the rifles from his men, ordered fire to be opened. Some 18 women were killed. Others were killed in disturbances elsewhere. In several cases the tribesmen had gathered ready to loot, when, as they expected, the women had driven the whites away.[46]

The women's participation was presumed by colonial officials and by journalists covering the story to be auxiliary to the actions of the real agents behind the rioting, Igbo men.

Neither the *Daily Herald* nor the *Manchester Guardian* mentioned that the rioters had been women, though both reported on Shiels' statement before parliament that women had been killed in the unrest. The *Daily Mail* did, indeed, note more prominently the participation of women. The *Daily Worker* wrote of the "massacre of African Women by the British Government" in January 1930, but, like the mainstream press, did not specify that the protesters were exclusively women. Rather, according to the paper, the rioters were "small peasants."[47] The *Daily Telegraph's* single article on the riots in December did not say a word about women at all. The *Woman's Leader*, a feminist paper affiliated with the National Union of Societies for Equal Citizenship, did not report on the riots. Only the *Morning Post*, under the headline "NATIVE RIOTS IN

NIGERIA. A Dozen Women Shot. Troops Repel Mass Attacks," observed that "a curious feature of the agitation was the fact that it was fomented by women, who organised mass attacks on certain small Government buildings and the treasury House." It then went on to say that "orders were apparently given to the troops to fire over the heads of the crowds," enabling the reader to assume that while women "fomented" the disturbances and were killed by troops trying to quell them, they did not constitute the entirety of the "mob."[48] The *African World*, a London weekly directed toward commercial and financial elites, initially carried the reports issued by Reuters, which repeated the information given out by the Colonial Office, though on 11 January 1930, it included a letter from its Lagos correspondent that sympathetically tied the rioting to women suffering from economic pressure. Buried in the fifth paragraph of a six-paragraph column, the correspondent asserted that in response to new efforts to tax the populace,

> women all over the districts rose up to protest against the system of utterly impoverishing them. Banks and other mercantile houses were broken into and their books and other materials damaged. Native Courts, which have become, in popular opinion, fattening houses for chiefs, were broken into and excesses committed. Further, it must be wrong to expect illiterate women, especially when infuriated, to understand and appreciate why they pay more for what they purchase from European stores while at the same time only the lowest prices is paid for produce.

The following week, the periodical observed that "in one place no less than twenty thousand women assembled and refused to disperse, but eventually were cleared out with sticks. Subsequently they returned, and it was then necessary to fire upon them." But the writer also tried to downplay the significance and unprecedented nature of the events, claiming that "the movement was neither political nor anti-foreign, and arose partly from a misunderstanding and partly at the instigation of some of the men."[49]

Press reports emanating from Nigeria later in 1930 carried more complete information about the women's war and gave it the significance it had received in official circles both in Nigeria and in London. A letter to *The Spectator* magazine of 24 May 1930, by "A Woman Correspondent," explicitly referred to the unrest as a "woman's rising" and noted its extraordinary scope and nature. She described the events of December 1929 as "the recent rising of some thousands of women out here; the first feminist movement in the modern manner, which extended over some hundreds of miles and included in an amazing way women of different districts and dialects who at ordinary times have apparently scarcely any communication with one another."[50]

Once the report of the commission of inquiry, which found that the shootings of women had been unjustified, was released in August, the press became more accurate in its accounts of the riots. On 25 August 1930, *The Times'* story by "a Nigerian Correspondent" asserted that

the trouble was of a nature and extent unprecedented in Nigeria. In a country where the women throughout the centuries have remained in subjection to the men, this was essentially a women's movement, organized, developed, and carried out by the women of the country, without either the help or permission of their menfolk, though probably with their tacit sympathy. The casualties resulting from the conflicts with the armed forces of the Crown were almost entirely women. Fifty-four were killed or died of wounds, and 57 were wounded. One man was accidentally killed and another wounded. The area involved was practically the whole of the two provinces, in extent larger than the six northernmost counties of England, containing a population of 2,750,000; and apart from the large numbers of armed police, nine companies of infantry had to be drafted into the area from other parts of Nigeria to complete the pacification of the disturbed area . . . . within three weeks of what they believed to be the first overt action by Government agents in the taxation of women numerous meetings had been held, the women's organizations were fully operative, and tens of thousands of women were demonstrating throughout the two provinces.[51]

The *Morning Post's* account quoted a local businessman who had observed "about 12,000 native women, some of them congregating from places almost 100 miles away, invad[ing] Aba to complain to the district officer about the reported intentions of the Government to impose a direct tax on the women." The paper noted that

the most interesting feature of the riots was the fact that they had been organised almost entirely by women in a community which was anything but a matriarchy. The men had been excluded from the meetings of the women, but they had given them their tacit support, and had accompanied them in war canoes on the occasion of their mass deputation to Aba. It was necessary to remember, however, that the women held great influence as they were largely the traders of the community.[52]

The *Daily Worker* entitled its coverage of the release of the report "Massacre of 54 Armed Women," and clearly stated that the risings in December 1929 had been the work of women who had "organised themselves in tens of thousands throughout the provinces."[53]

Public response to the press coverage, even when it succeeded in conveying the extraordinary nature, scope, and significance of the women's war, seems to have been almost non-existent. No letters to the editor appeared in the major dailies. Members of parliament restricted their questions, for the most part, to matters of information-gathering; they made no protest against the actions of the troops until 29 January 1930, when Mr. Kedward asked Shiels "whether, during the recent disturbances in Nigeria, machine guns were used to fire upon the women in Etim Ekpo and Abak; and, if so, what action he propose[d] to take in the matter?" When Shiels replied that at Abak "shots had been fired by the police, who are not armed with machine guns, and at Utu Etim Ekpo the number of casualties was four," Kedward appears not to have noticed Shiels' failure to answer his question, and proceeded to question the Undersecretary of State for the Colonies about the collective punishment imposed on the villages of southeast Nigeria. This latter issue seemed to exercise Kedward and other MPs far more than the shooting of the women did.[54] When the report of the second commission of inquiry concluded that the shootings were unjustified, Mr. Horrabin demanded to know

> what action the Government proposes to take ... [and] whether the recommendations of the Aba commission of inquiry into the disturbances ... , particularly as regard the free pardon of certain persons, the desirability of changes in the methods of imposing taxation, and the reconsideration both of the collective fines actually imposed and of the whole subject of collective punishment, are being carried into effect?

"Can we," he asked wryly, "have some assurance that the officers responsible for these cases are at least being removed to areas which will give their qualities rather less scope?"[55]

That reassurance never arrived, but its absence provoked little public comment. On 27 January 1931, the Secretary of State for the Colonies, Lord Passfield, issued a dispatch to the Government of Nigeria regarding the Aba Riots and the report produced by the commission of inquiry into them. He declined to place blame on the officers involved in the shooting of the women and took no action against them. Horrabin questioned Shiels about the decision in parliament on 18 February 1931, but offered no objection when Shiels avowed that "no ground has been found for disciplinary action against the officers commanding the detachments of troops concerned."[56] The press was silent on the decision.

We need to ask why the women's actions and the killing of nearly 60 of them evoked no real reaction from the British at home. One explanation for the silence surrounding the women's war derives from the extraordinary, fantastic, and finally monstrous images of half-naked native women without their children, apparently dressed for war in palm fronds, alleged to be armed with machetes and cudgels, though they carried no more than sticks, and amassing suddenly in the thousands from seemingly out of nowhere. Passfield's exoneration of the soldiers who fired upon and killed women at Opobo and Utu Etim Ekpo argued that

> the situations with which the various officers were confronted were without precedent, so far as I can judge, I might almost say in the history of the British Empire. Disturbances in which women have taken the foremost, or the only part, are not unknown here and elsewhere in the Empire, but administrative, policy, and military officers in Nigeria could hardly anticipate demonstrations by hundreds, or even thousands, of native women ... developing, in some cases at any rate, into definite attacks on the property of Government or of private individuals; and in some cases threatening life.

British officers and officials found it impossible to believe that such behavior and coordinated action could have been undertaken by the women alone, and insisted, both implicitly, as we have seen in press accounts, and explicitly, that their menfolk were behind the whole thing, putting their women forward in the belief that the British would not fire on them. Witnesses before the inquest and the commission of inquiry repeatedly volunteered that the women's actions were unlike any they had seen before. To the British officers and colonial officials, the women's dress and demeanor conjured up mythic images of powerful and frightening women. "We are liable to forget that the King of Dahomey's Amazon bodyguard was not a fiction," noted J.E.W. Flood in a memorandum to A. Fiddian, "and if a howling mob of excited female savages who would be quite ready to tear a man in pieces with their hands is about the place, the only thing to do is to take strong action." Indeed, as a number of early reports indicated, British officials and officers feared that had the African women not been stopped by gunfire at Opobo, "probably the entire European and loyal population [would have been] massacred." What the British described as wild, frenzied, howling, menacing, frantically excited, gesticulating, lawless, savage, ferocious mobs of bare-breasted women obviously could not have fit into any possible category of womanhood recognizable to the men, and left only the realm of the fantastic in which to place them and their actions.[57]

But as we have seen, the imagery of mobs of women overwhelming male defenses was not limited to African women in the fall of 1929. When asked by a commission member whether "you would not have acted in the same way had you been among the suffragettes in England," D.O. Whitman replied, "There is no comparison at all."[58] But the testimony of one African woman, Ahudi of Nsidimo, before the Aba commission, may have suggested that such a comparison might indeed be apt, that British women may have certain shared or common interests with the women of the *Ògù Umùnwaànyi*. Ahudi warned the commission, "unless you come to a conclusion which will satisfy the women, we will follow you wherever you go. Formerly we never made demonstrations in this manner, but we do so now in order to show you that women are annoyed... No doubt there are women like ourselves in your country. If need be we will write to them to help us".[59]

The forces that threatened to disintegrate, even to annihilate the subject,[60] manifested themselves in the behavior and actions of the Nigerian women who rose up against British authorities in 1929. It may be that the images required to process the threat—images found not in the world of the real as westerners understood it, but images conjured from the realm of the pre-conscious symbolic of fantastic, mythic, monstrous women with the power to overwhelm and dissolve the vulnerable, shattered subject of the interwar period—posed such a threat to individual and collective psychic survival that they had to be destroyed. The fantasies, fears, and anxieties conjured up by the actions of the women involved prevented them from being assimilated in an ordinary conscious way. Unable, literally, to take them in, to articulate or represent them in intelligible terms, Britons simply did not. The events of the women's war may also have threatened to re-open the traumas of Amritsar, a possibility that could not be contemplated, especially not after an election in which women under 30 had participated for the first time and had returned a government regarded by many members of society as the handmaidens of bolshevism. The possibility of the conflation of "flappers" with the threatening figures of the women's war, however unconsciously made, cannot be dismissed. Traumatized nations, like traumatized people, sometimes must "forget" certain incidents or events, "especially," notes Larry Ray, "where the past poses a threat to the unity of the nation."[61] "Mass forgetting," and even outright denials of cultural traumas are part of the arsenal societies, like individuals, use to defend against the dissolution that these terrifying events might bring about.[62] Recovery from the war that had called forth these terrors in the first instance required destroying the threatening women of southeastern Nigeria and domesticating those at home.

Conclusion: Resolving the "National Crisis" of 1929–1931

> Until now the class-mania more than anything else has prevented this nation's recovery from the War.[1]
> The Parliamentary Labour Party had been not defeated but annihilated: largely we think by the women's vote.[2]

When Labour took office again in October 1929, it faced severe challenges in virtually every aspect of national life—unemployment, finance, international affairs, colonial policy, and political instability at home. Disruption of the international financial markets, as London ceded its supremacy to New York; dislocation of industry and trade, both at home and abroad; struggles over disarmament among the great powers; sharpening nationalist sentiments in the colonies; and the apparent failure of the three-party system to provide effective government—all of them aftershocks of the Great War—gave rise in 1930 to the conviction that Britain faced a "crisis" of grave proportions. In part a reflection of the real problems facing the country, in part a device mobilized in the hope of discrediting the Labour government and effecting a change in political power and policies, the "national crisis," described by one historian in 1992 as "the greatest peacetime crisis in Britain this century," transformed the political landscape in Britain.[3]

Labour came into power as a minority government, dependent upon the Liberals for their majority, just as the economy, responding to the deepening worldwide depression, took a sharp downward turn. British exports, amounting to £839 million in 1929, dropped to £666 million in 1930, and to £461M in 1931. Figures for those who were out of work registered the declining economic fortunes of the country: the number of unemployed reached 1.520 million in January 1930, 1.761 million in April, 2,070 million in July, 2.319 million in October, and

180

2.5 million in December 1930. The Labour government squandered any chances it might have had to alleviate the economic distress by introducing measures no more vigorous in their vision or execution than their Conservative predecessors. Its limited commitment to public works programs did little to dent the severity of the downturn, and the government would not support more dramatic measures to stimulate the economy. It did introduce the Unemployment Insurance bill in November 1929, increasing the numbers of those who could get relief without having made sufficient contributions to the fund and thereby placing a larger draw on the Treasury. The bill became law in 1930.

Internationally, despite truly heroic efforts by MacDonald and Foreign Secretary Arthur Henderson, efforts to promote peace proceeded unevenly. In 1929, the Young Plan had restructured German reparations and provided for the evacuation of the Rhineland by allied troops in 1930. But Foreign Minister Streseman was dead by the time Labour took office, and with him the prospects of German efforts toward lasting peace. The cut-off of foreign capital to Germany in 1930 caused its artificially prosperous economy to falter; the need for budget cuts provoked unrest, and led Bruening, the German chancellor, to invoke emergency powers. In the election in September, the National Socialist party won 107 seats in the Reichstag, an increase of 97 from its previous showing. In Italy in May, Mussolini trumpeted his preference for "rifles, machine-guns, warships, aeroplanes, and cannon" over "words." And although Britain, the United States, and Japan agreed at the London Naval Conference in April 1930 to limit the size of their fleets, neither Italy nor France would sign on to the treaty, thus vitiating its effectiveness. Problems in the Mideast flared with the failure of treaty negotiations with Egypt and troubles between Arabs and Jews in Palestine. In the empire, revolt in Nigeria, the second most important colony, elicited sufficient concern among the permanent members of the Colonial Office, if not among the politicians or the country as a whole, to bring about substantial change in the way the British would rule there.

Events in India caused serious discomfort for the country. The massacre at Amritsar had inflamed nationalist opinion, sparking disorder throughout the 1920s. In 1927, Baldwin's government had established a commission headed by Sir John Simon to assess the efficacy of the 1919 Montagu-Chelmsford reforms; lacking any Indian representation, it aroused only suspicion and disdain among Indian nationalists. In October 1929, Lord Irwin, the Viceroy, declared that "the natural issue of India's constitutional progress ... is the attainment of Dominion status," infuriating Conservatives but underwhelming members of the Indian

Congress party, which in December of that year issued a "declaration of independence," in pursuit of which it launched a boycott of central and provincial governments and a campaign of civil disobedience, including non-payment of taxes.[4] When the Simon Commission released its report calling for an enlarged Indian electorate, more self-government in the provinces, and a conference to decide the shape of the future central government in June 1930, its measures became lost in the turmoil of Gandhi's civil disobedience campaign. He and a number of Congress party leaders had been jailed, as had some 54,000 other participants in the campaign, whose arrests, the Indian government hoped, would curtail the disorder. MacDonald did convene the first of three Round Table conferences in London in November 1930 to discuss the future of India's government, though Congress party members refused to attend it. When the government approached the Conservative party in January 1931 for its support for further discussions about a new constitution for India, which it received, Churchill could not contain his fury, and resigned from the Conservative shadow cabinet. (The second Round Table Conference met in the fall of 1931, by which time the Labour government had given way to the National government, in which Churchill was conspicuous by his absence.)

Talk of a "national crisis" erupted in the fall of 1930 after months of public perseverating about Britain's precarious state. In June 1930, for instance, Churchill delivered the Romanes lecture, in which he characterized "these eventful years through which we are passing" as "not less serious for us than the years of the Great War...We see our race doubtful of its mission and no longer confident about its principles, infirm of purpose, drifting to and fro with the tides and currents of a deeply-disturbed ocean." His language, recalling both the war and the imagery of swamping we have seen in previous chapters, should alert us to the fact that the crisis of boundaries created by trauma had not slackened over the decade. Across all shades of political opinion, among virtually every section of public life, the idea of a national crisis approaching war-time levels took hold, fed by conviction and opportunism alike. MacDonald and Lloyd George spoke of it as the worst situation facing the country since "the darkest hours of the War."[5] The *Daily Mail* used the occasion offered by the Bank Holiday of 3 August to recall the other Bank Holiday in 1914, "immediately preceding the war," which "inevitably recalls thoughts of what happened seventeen years ago."

So fearful was the conflict and so grievous were the wounds which it inflicted that we are still suffering from its aftermath. Yesterday's anniversary finds us with problems of the gravest character to face and solve. They are the direct legacy of the war, and they cannot be shirked. To shirk them would be at one and the same time to betray those who gave their lives and to ruin ourselves.[6]

The foreign and domestic difficulties facing Britain seemed beyond the ability of the political parties to manage. Labour, we have seen, did not by itself hold sufficient seats to govern; it depended upon Liberal support to stay in office. Internally, the party faced significant dissent from its left wing. Conservatives faced their own internal strife: Baldwin came under attack first by Lord Beaverbrook and then by Lord Rothermere and Churchill over issues of imperial free trade and dominion status for India. He survived those assaults, and actually emerged stronger for them, but the public bloodletting did nothing to boost the confidence of the nation in the ability of its political leaders. Newspaper editors questioned the competence and capabilities of politicians; politicians themselves worried about the public's "disillusionment" with parliamentary government and noted that conditions in Britain were not dissimilar to those in other countries that had turned to dictatorship. Ordinary party politics, it appeared to more and more people, could not continue in this vein. The king's secretary, Lord Stamfordham, wrote to MacDonald in October 1930 that "the time has come when even emergency measures may be necessary to avert a calamity which...is not altogether incomparable with the Great War." As historian Philip Williamson has observed, public momentum for a new approach to government was building rapidly.[7]

Sir Oswald Mosley, Labour minister and ex-soldier who believed himself to represent the "war generation," thought he saw his chance. Disdainful of the failure of Labour to take effective control of the situation, he proposed a series of policies designed to deal with unemployment and economic stagnation through state planning of trade, industry, and finance. When the cabinet rebuffed him, he resigned his position and began to reach out to others who shared his conviction that dangerous times called for "ruthless Realism," "soaring Idealism," and decisive "action." Luminaries from across the political spectrum— Churchill, John Maynard Keynes, Lord Rothermere, J.L. Garvin of the *Observer*, Harold Nicolson, Lord Beaverbrook, Lloyd George, A.J. Cook, and the Astors—expressed interest in and support for some of his ideas, though they did not go so far as to join his New party when he formed it in March 1931. The fact that his program could command the attention and respect of such an array of serious people illustrates the degree to which conventional politics had fallen into disrepute.

Economic and financial conditions worsened during the spring and summer of 1931, culminating in the crisis that brought down the Labour government on 23 August. Unemployment reached 2.707 million by June, leading the government to seek parliamentary approval for an increase in borrowing power for the unemployment insurance fund. The Committee on National Expenditure, formed in February 1931 under the leadership of Sir George May, issued its report on 31 July; it predicted a deficit of £120 million by April 1932 and called for new taxes of £24 million and cuts of £96 million to meet it. Cuts totaling £66.6 million, the report recommended, should come from unemployment benefits. The May report brought home to Britain the financial crisis that had rippled through the international financial system throughout the spring and summer, as skittish foreign investors, leery that a beleaguered Labour government could make such deep cuts, began to withdraw their funds; the drain on the banks continued well into August. Bankers demanded action on the part of the government to renew confidence in the pound by balancing the budget.

The draconian nature of these cuts, it became clear to many opinion-makers, were beyond the capacity of any party to introduce. "No single party can attempt to do a third of what the Committee recommends," wrote Garvin on 2 August 1931, "Labour would be broken to bits by the attempt. Liberalism, if an accessory, would be annihilated. Only a National Government with all parties implicated in the responsibility can hope to grapple with the tremendous problems of public finance."[8] Cabinet officials did not dispute the need to balance the budget; they differed over the amount of cuts that would have to be made to the unemployment benefit. The cabinet's Economy Committee announced on 13 August that it would balance the budget through "equality of sacrifice," acknowledging that some of the deficit would have to be made up from the unemployment insurance fund. When it became clear to a number of cabinet ministers ten days later, however, that these cuts would be substantial, they opposed the budget plan. With a cabinet split of 11 to 9, members agreed on 22 August to resign immediately and inform the king of their decision; they recommended that he convene a conference of MacDonald, Baldwin, and Herbert Samuel (serving as leader of the Liberal party in the absence of Lloyd George owing to illness) to determine how power would be transferred. When he returned the next day MacDonald informed his cabinet colleagues, to their "utter stupefaction," as one historian described it,[9] that a National government made up of Conservatives, Liberals, and Labour—with he himself as prime minister—would succeed the Labour government. It would consist of four Labourites, four Conservatives, and two Liberals. Upon hearing of the plan from her husband, who had served in the Labour government, Beatrice Webb commented in her diary on 24 August 1931, "British credit may be temporarily saved but internal peace is jeopardised for many a long year."[10] Events would prove her wrong.

A temporary government of individuals, not parties, it was believed, could best meet the financial crisis that gripped the country, which would necessitate cuts and tax increases too great for any government based on party to make and still remain in power. Fears of class resentment that might "align party politics on lines of class warfare for 20 years," as Liberal Lord Lothian cautioned, informed discussions, underscoring the conviction of National government ministers that shared, "equitable sacrifices" imposed on the "nation" would be the only way to resolve the crisis. The budget measure that resulted required retrenchment in the area of unemployment insurance, but it also entailed (sometimes considerable) salary reductions for civil servants and higher taxes on middle-level income earners. These latter suffered perhaps the greatest sacrifice; the wealthy certainly were required to pay higher taxes but their burden did not match that put on the middle classes, proportionately speaking. The apparent "national" nature of the cuts and tax increases enabled the Conservative and Liberal parties to debate the measure in the House as representatives of a national coalition rather than representatives of class interest. Labour MPs could be cast as an "irresponsible" opposition to the "national" good.[11]

The government was to sit for six weeks only and an election fought by the parties was to be held to replace it with a conventional party government. The response of the Labour party and the TUC to the budget, however, forced the National government to reconsider that decision. Led by Arthur Henderson, George Lansbury, and TUC leaders Ernest Bevin and J.R. Clynes, the Labour party turned to a program far more frankly "socialist" in nature. No longer constrained by the need to be regarded as trustworthy or fit to govern through their accommodation with other parties, Labour party members put forward ideas of state control over industry, banking, and finance, a platform, Conservatives and Liberals feared, that would have great appeal to the public, making it impossible for any new government to continue on a course designed to sustain confidence in the financial markets and address the problems of the economy. If Labour were to win the election on the basis of promises to restore the cuts, another financial crisis would undoubtedly arise, causing sterling to collapse and the economy to take a nosedive. "Not just financial and economic stability, but also political and social stability seemed to be at stake," Williamson has asserted.[12] For, beginning in mid-September, public opposition to the budget cuts began to appear, some of it from quarters entirely unexpected by the government.

Authorities had no difficulty dealing with marches and demonstrations on the part of the unemployed; they cast these protests as issues of law and order. They had less success dismissing the objections from teachers and from judges, whose effectiveness at oratory and argumentation served their causes well. But the most serious opposition arose within the Atlantic fleet, stationed at Invergordon for naval exercises, when on 15 September 1931, sailors—hit by cuts in their salaries— refused orders to set sail. By the next day, authorities had lost control of the situation. Fearful that repressive measures would simply ratchet up instances of indiscipline, the Admiralty cancelled the exercises, dispersed the fleet, and announced a decision to postpone cuts in pay until they could be re-examined. The implication that they might be reversed after such an examination appears to have convinced the men to stand down from their positions. A mutiny this was not, as the Admiralty recognized, but this kind of action on the part of naval crews, members of the most exalted branch of the armed services, had a significant impact on political leaders. By the beginning of October, the cabinet had announced that it would fight the next election, set for 27 October, as a National party, a decision that, apart from pulling the rug out from under Mosley's once-promising prospects of a viable national alternative in his New party, "shattered the pattern of politics" in Britain, as Williamson has observed.[13] Putting the fractured and fragmented political body back together in a new national configuration would have the effect of repairing the fractured psyche of the nation as well, restoring a perceived unity and wholeness that had been shattered by the traumas of the Great War.

Labour leaders, stunned by MacDonald's decision to head a national government in August, were disgusted by his choice to lead an election against the party, a breach so grievous that they gave up any lingering loyalties they might have had to him and pursued their newly aggressive agenda with a zeal unhampered by regret or sympathy for the man who had led them for so long. At their October conference, party members and TUC delegates produced a program that made it clear that Labour would never again be, in Beatrice Webb's words, "the caretaker of the existing order of society." In an election manifesto written up by Harold Laski, the party promised not only to restore the cuts in benefits but to nationalize the banks and credit systems, coal mines, power, transport, iron and steel, and land, making provisions for worker participation in the management of these publicly-owned industries. Philip Snowden, who had remained with MacDonald in the National government, denounced the Labour program as "the most fantastic and impracticable ever put before the electors." "This is not Socialism," he sputtered over the BBC airways. "It is bolshevism run mad."[14]

It was against bolshevism run mad that the National parties organized for the October election. Success depended upon discipline in putting forward a single candidate against the Labour candidate in each constituency; three-way races involving a Liberal, a Conservative, and a Labourite would only split the vote and hand the election to Labour. In constituencies formerly contested by both Conservatives and Liberals, one dropped out, leaving Labour candidates to face a single opponent. In this way, the partners in the National coalition, including the National Labour members under MacDonald, Thomas, and Snowden, fashioned themselves into a self-conscious and "massive anti-socialist electoral force," resolving to end the threat of socialism once and for all. "The great thing this time," confided Baldwin in a moment of indiscretion, "is to give Socialism a really smashing defeat."[15]

Once plans for the new election, to be held in late October 1931, were announced, the allusions to the Great War that had characterized talk of the "national crisis" in August resumed with an incredible intensity. Casting the economic and financial crises as a "national emergency" that had necessitated a government that could represent the nation as a whole rather than sectional or class interests enabled politicians, newspaper editors, business and trade organizations, writers, and church leaders to portray the TUC and the Labour party as unpatriotic. The *Observer*, whose editor, J.L. Garvin, enjoyed the respect of a wide variety of political opinion, had, from the moment the May report was issued at the end of July, beaten the drum of war-talk incessantly, casting Labour and socialism as enemies of the people no less dangerous than Germany had been. In an editorial written the day before the National government was formed, the *Observer* described the parties as being caught in "barbed wire entanglements." The next edition applauded the formation of the National government under MacDonald; "with his eyes wide open to risks as extreme as any national war leader ever yet ran in time of peace," the paper gushed, "he faced them without doubting or flinching like a man of men." It approved entirely of Baldwin and

Neville Chamberlain taking up seats in the cabinet, assuring them that "if they trust to the power of patriotism, if they recall the memories of the War, if they appeal for sacrifice in the spirit of war-time, they will be backed by their party to a man and a woman." The National government would need that kind of wartime support, for the next election, it warned, "will be in itself another crisis as dangerous as war." "Every citizen must understand that we are at the beginning of a life-and-death business and that nothing but a supreme exertion of patriotism can avail...the fate of Britain will swing in the scales. That and nothing less is going to be the issue—revival or ruin."[16]

The language mobilized by National government adherents echoed that of wartime accounts. Were Labour to prevail, for example, "the world's confidence in the future of British finance and credit would be shattered for good. And beyond any doubt whatever Britain, self undone, would become the most irretrievably defeated nation amongst all the belligerents who fought in the World-War." MacDonald wrote to his constituency at the Seaham Labour party meeting that "we have to face the question of how to meet that crisis or allow it to come upon us and shatter us." Every week the *Observer* sounded its alarm, ultimately portraying the crisis not simply as *like* the war, but as a continuation of it. One essay by Garvin declared that

> we have now only a limited time to decide whether we shall recover from the War or shall never recover.... The question is whether Britain alone shall fail to recover from the War—whether all that has made the greatness of this island and this breed is to pass away—whether irretrievable Defeat at a second remove is to be the real sequel of all our efforts in the War, and to write the last epitaph of our dead—whether class shall overcome country—whether ignorance, faction, and mass-bribery within the gates shall be more fatal at last than any foreign enemy.[17]

Victory and recovery—even existence itself—depended upon the nation choosing patriotism over class war; Labour's repudiation of the former had nearly brought the country to its knees, the *Observer* declared. "Whatever they say now, most of them with respect to patriotism have thought little and one less. In patriotism there is a guiding, unifying, and saving power which nothing yet known can replace. Until now the class-mania more than anything else has prevented this nation's recovery from the War." Meeting the present crisis would require "a strong race with the moral grit of war-time." Only a National government could provide the patriotism, the unity that would enable the people to face Britain's "life-and-death" predicament. The "necessity—as urgent, as imperative, in this state of peace as it ever was in the War—is National government on the broadest practicable basis."[18]

Labour had betrayed the nation in its refusal to face the economic crisis in August; their actions had weakened Britain's stability and infected the country with "class-spirit instead of national discipline which they had spread until it reach the very fleet." Voters must recognize that "Britain's fate is as strictly staked as ever it was in war. We have to grapple at home with peril of a kind which, if not now crushed at the polls with a moral strength never to be forgotten, will prove more fatal than any foreign enemy." In fact, the paper alleged, Labour's actions had already threatened international peace by fomenting the resistance of the sailors at Invergorden. Without a "strong and solvent Britain" the world could not maintain stability. "The lowering of her name since the troubles in the Fleet is a universal peril, as the Manchurian situation makes plain," alluding to Japan's incursion into Chinese territory. Referring to Labour as "the nation-wreckers" and castigating its "program of bankruptcy and disintegration," the paper urged that a Labour victory would result in "a denationalised and suicidal democracy in whom no trust can be placed." The country would be annihilated, the "splendour of our effort in the War" wasted. "Vote to fulfil somewhat the dream of the men who meant to die for something better than this," it urged, in a rehearsal of the worn-out ideal of a home fit for heroes.[19]

Virtually all the other national newspapers repeated the themes of war, patriotism, and the enemies of the nation. In a clear formulation of those who sought to destroy the nation and those who would fight tooth and nail to defend it, Churchill, in a piece in the *Daily Mail*, referred to "the loyal forces in every street and village," as against "the subversive forces" led by Labour. "Never," he then assured readers, "apart from war-time, were those strong forces which have made Britain what she is more united at heart...or more ready to follow valiant and faithful leadership." The *Daily Express* issued "A Warning to M.P.s" that Labour would return from its party congress "to attack and destroy the Administration in every possible way." It exulted that the October election would "end for ever the status of Great Britain as a crumbling European State. This election must begin, instead, the glorious story of a united Empire.... The British Empire will stand as an indestructible rock against the tempests of disorder and disorganisation." Were the Labour party to win, it charged, in a piece subtitled, "Is it Peace or War?" "the forces of disruption will be let loose in every country. The markets of the world will be swept by panic. Currencies will begin their mad St. Vitus's dance once more. Bolshevism will burst its barriers."[20] Once again we hear echoes of boundary-crossing too intolerable to contemplate.

In an article entitled "Is England Worth Saving?" Philip Gibbs compared the current perilous situation to the March 1918 spring offensive of Germany. "To-morrow such a day is coming again," he intoned, "when our safety as a nation, our place in the world, and our chance of decent prosperity depend on the spirit of our folk." "To-morrow I shall vote for a National Government because it promises a truce to party politics for the nation's sake," he told his audience, and in a formulation reflecting the earlier re-writing of the General Strike that brought workers—though not their political leaders—back into the national fold and echoed the representation of the crisis as one very like if not actually warfare, Gibbs reminded readers that "our young men of to-day who came out—on both sides—during the general strike of 1926 showed that they had the same grit as their elder brothers who went singing down the Bapaume road." *The Times* carried an appeal from the Archbishop of Canterbury and the Federal Council of the Evangelical Free Churches of England urging Britons to vote for the National government slate so as to uphold "the welfare of the country." It, too, made the comparison to the Great War in a bid to remind voters of the gravity of the situation.

> At the season of commemoration of the Armistice we shall pray that we may worthily take our part in the establishment of true peace throughout the world, and also that, remembering the sacrifice offered by our brethren for their country and ours, we may be ready to bear the sacrifice which it asks of us in an hour of different, but not less real need.

The *Daily Mail* editorialized on the eve of the election that "if you vote for the National Government you will rescue your country from a peril even deadlier than any which menaced her in the war. If, on the other hand, you return the Socialists or give an indecisive verdict, you seal her fate for ever and bring unutterable ruin on yourselves." "Vote To-day to Save the Nation and Yourself," urged the election-day headline. "A wrong choice," the paper thundered in an unusually bald reference to annihilation, "and the consequences will be national death." Finally, it expressed its faith that the voters of Britain would come through: "they will, in fact, repeat in peace what our soldiers achieved in those desperate hours of the war when the enemy offensives threatened destruction and the British armies fought with their 'backs to the wall.' England conquered then, and she will conquer now."[21]

Only the *Daily Herald* and the Manchester *Guardian* refrained from resorting to the over-heated rhetoric about the nation under attack from its enemies, the *Herald* turning the language of nation against the National government parties in a bid to show up the class and sectional interests of its leaders. It ridiculed the idea that a government purporting to act patriotically on behalf of the nation should submit to the demands of international bankers to impose benefit cuts on unemployed Britons.

> Where is the patriotism, we may ask, in allowing the Federal Reserve Bank of New York to dictate, as the condition for a further credit to the Bank of England, the policy to be pursued in relation to unemployment benefit? This is not patriotism, but acceptance of the dictatorship not even of a British bank, but of international finance,

the paper argued. In an editorial titled "On Being British," the *Herald* declared that by choosing to first reduce the salaries of civil servants, teachers, and police and cut unemployment benefits, the National government could not lay claim to acting on behalf of the nation. "Is this British?" it asked, and answered, "No." "No part of the national burden should be placed on shoulders unable to bear it," the paper declared, and claimed that in protecting the unemployed, the Labour party "has been British."[22]

Beginning in early October, the *Herald* ran editorials to expose National government claims to represent the nation as shameful and divisive. In an article entitled "Who is the 'Nation'?" the paper protested "Our 'Nationalists'...insolent...device...of arrogating to themselves the claim to speak for and on behalf of 'the nation,' to represent 'the nation,' to be 'the nation.' To oppose them is, they would persuade people, to oppose 'the nation,' to be guilty of something verging on high treason." The paper decried the unprecedented and unparalleled "attempt to divide the nation into the 'two nations' of which Disraeli wrote, to class one of them as helots, as outlanders, as men and women beyond the pale." It castigated the government's creation of the "pretence of a united 'National Party' arrayed against a 'national enemy.'" So far from being a "national enemy," the paper insisted, claiming the "national" mantle for the party of the working classes,

Labour stands for the reorganisation of the financial, industrial and
economic system of the nation, on which not only its prosperity
but its very life depend. It stands for the subordination of private
vested interests to the national need. It stands for the defence of the
standard of living of the workers and for the maintenance of those
social services which are their national heritage. It stands for a sound
finance which will neither plunder the poor nor increase the tribute
levied upon the nation by a class.

In standing against the National government, behind whose camou-
flage the Tories were able to act according to their true colors, Labour
"is the guardian of the welfare and of the interests of the vast majority
of the people of this country. It is performing a national duty."[23]

As election day drew near, the *Herald* pulled out all the stops. Asserting
that "the whole fundamental system of democracy is at issue," George
Lansbury painted the National government and its supporters as fascist
in their efforts to capture the electorate. "The insistent claim of a Party to
represent the nation," he insisted, "the denunciation of all opponents as
enemies of the State; the arrogant pretension that the safety of the realm
is dependent on the retention of office by its present holders; all these
things are of the essence of Fascism." "A vote for the 'Nationals'," he
warned, "is a vote against democracy, a vote against political freedom, a
vote for the pinchbeck Fascism of a bunch of pinchbeck Mussolinis."[24]

In the event, the country voted overwhelmingly on 27 October 1931
for the return of the National government. Having been convinced
of a "national crisis" that only a "national government" representing
"national unity" could address and resolve, voters gave National government candidates 67 percent of their votes in "the greatest British
election victory of modern times, greatly surpassing even that of 1918."
Of the 615 members of parliament who would take their seats, 554 of
them would be members of the National government party, giving them
a majority of over 500.[25]

The election proved devastating for the Labour party. Of the 267 seats
it had held, it lost 215 of them, leaving a party of only 46 MPs in the
House of Commons. As Williamson has pointed out, this "was even
fewer than after the party's first attempt to become a major political
force, in 1918."[26] It had, to be sure, maintained and even, in some
places, increased its popular vote, but its majorities occurred only in
some locations, certainly not in enough constituencies to establish the
party as any kind of electoral threat. The victory of the National government reclaimed for the nation, it seemed, the last of those forces

that seemed to have disturbed it, women. Beatrice Webb remarked about the election, in language to which we have become so accustomed, that "the Parliamentary Labour Party had been not defeated but annihilated: largely we think by the women's vote."[27] The *Observer* concurred, telling its readers that an influx of new voters had helped save the day. "Amongst these new reinforcements of the State," the paper declared, "most were women. Their franchise has been justified by their instinct. Many of them in working-class constituencies voted dead against the males in their own households."[28]

The *Observer* spoke of "The electoral massacre of ex-Ministers," while the *Daily Express* carried the front page banner, "Socialist Party Wiped Out." The *Daily Mail* trumpeted its headline, "Socialist Party Shattered at the Polls," in the language of the traumatized, but this time displacing the fears of the victors onto the vanquished. "This election is the sign," it followed up the next day, "that the tide of Socialism, which has risen steadily for a century, has begun to ebb."[29] The paper appears to have it right; Labour MP Morgan Philips Price complained to Charles Trevelyan that the victory of the National government was "an English form of a Fascist coup d'etat," an observation echoed, surprisingly, by Conservative leaders. Neville Chamberlain called it a "bloodless [but] ... none the less effective ... political revolution" which had produced a "Parliamentary Dictatorship." Conservative party chairman J.C.C. Davidson told William Davidson on 5 November 1931 that "in effect the British nation has done through the ballot box what Continental countries can only do by revolution. We have a Dictatorship."[30]

Britons had not, of course, elected a fascist government; in fact, this book argues, organized fascism in Britain did not take hold in the same way it did in Italy or Germany because an English version of what might be called a fascistic sensibility had already been established by the early 1920s. Although they commanded a good deal of attention in the 1930s and even, for a short time, attracted the support of establishment Britons like Lord Rothermere, blackshirted fascists held limited appeal, because the ideas about alien "others" they sought to put forward were redundant: those ideas had been accepted by various political groups of the right and left already and the British Union of Fascists offered little that could be considered new. Whatever else it had done, the election of 1931 had undoubtedly forged a "nation." The overwhelming victory of the National government over the Labour opposition enabled the country to displace its fears of being swamped, overcome by invading forces, by projecting them on to those who had been defeated. Fears of annihilation were put away through the annihilation of the enemy. "Had we failed to return a strong National Government, had we enthroned Socialism in the seat of power, the forces of discouragement and disruption would have broken their bounds and overflowed the nation," exclaimed the *Daily Express*. "A policy making for bankruptcy, class-hate, disintegration, and the fall of our land for ever, has been smashed, pulverised, and annihilated by the vote of a free democracy," proclaimed the *Observer*. "After last week's verdict no future crisis can threaten in the same way the foundations of the State."[31]

The paper was not far off the mark. When the abdication crisis of Edward VIII in 1936—discussion of which in public and private explicitly took place in the context of fears about fascism—threw up the possibility of "real" dictatorship in the form of a "King's Party," behind which Mosley, Churchill, and Lord Beaverbrook threw their support, the country as a whole decisively turned away from any manifestation of it. The Labour party had recovered a fair portion of its electoral support and had achieved reintegration within the nation as the responsible opposition by the time the king's desire to marry Wallis Simpson triggered a behind-the-scenes confrontation with Baldwin's cabinet. The appearance of what cabinet minutes described as "a divergence between [the king] and his ministers" had provoked a Clydeside member of parliament to protest, "I see we are going to have a Fascist King, are we?"[32] Kingsley Martin, editor of the socialist-leaning *New Statesman and Nation*, reminded readers that "if we drop the trappings of Monarchy in the gutter, . . . Germany has taught us that some gutter-snipe (or house-painter with a mission) may pick them up."[33]

Determination to prevent any such possibility united the government and the Labour party. A summary of the "Attitude of the British Press" in the cabinet papers took pains to single out the *Daily Herald*, "the official organ of the Labour Party and of the Trade Unions," it pointed out, as having made "the principle contribution to the discussion of the constitutional side." The paper, noted the summary, while acknowledging the "personal sadness" of the situation for the king and Mrs. Simpson,

completely supports the Cabinet in the advice it has tendered and then . . . bluntly declares that only one reply is possible, i.e. either The King is bound to accept his Minister's advice or else the British democratic constitution ceases to work and the Nation is confronted with issues which go back to the constitutional struggles between Parliament and King of 250 years ago. Of all parties it declares Labour must be most sensitive to the constitutional implications of a dispute where the outcome has public consequences between the King and the Government which the people has freely chosen to represent it.

The author of this document emphasized Labour's "solid support" of the government a number of times; he noted "the fact that Members of the House and especially Labour members have returned... solidly behind the Government in the attitude it has taken throughout the period of crisis."[34]

The comparisons of the 1931 "national crisis" to the Great War allowed the economic, political, and social difficulties of the 1920s to stand in for the military conflict that had produced such horrors, so much loss and grief. And in resolving the crisis of the nation, as the *Observer* suggested, the traumas thrown up by the war could now be put to rest. "In that hour of trial," it stated with what seemed a sigh in relief, "we have kept the faith that those who died for it through the war-years charged us to keep."[35] In likening the national crisis to the Great War, and in resolving it by electing a National government, Britons created the narrative conditions necessary to bring their collective trauma to an end. Its resolution brought to a close the long national nightmare that had haunted the country since the end of the war, enabling Britain to emerge from its traumatized state and go forward, however ignominiously, into the new decade, its national identity established, the national psyche repaired and made whole.

Notes

Introduction

1. Charles Edmunds [pseudonym of Charles E. Carrington], *A Subaltern's War* (New York, 1930), p. 194.
2. Quoted in Alan Judd, *Ford Madox Ford* (Cambridge, Ma., 1990), p. 297; Ford Madox Ford, *Parade's End* (New York, 1979), pp. 659–660; Edmunds, *A Subaltern's War*, p. 113; W.N. Maxwell, *A Psychological Retrospect of the Great War* (London, 1923); Caroline E. Playne, *Society at War, 1914–1916* (Boston, 1931), p. 7; See also Caroline E. Playne, *Britain Holds On, 1917, 1918* (London, 1933); Philip Gibbs, *Heirs Apparent* (New York, 1924), p. 257; quoted in Trudi Tate, *Modernism, History and the First World War* (Manchester, 1998), p. 16.
3. Allan Young argues that PTSD "is not timeless, nor does it possess an intrinsic unity. Rather, it is glued together by the practices, technologies, and narratives with which it is diagnosed, studied, treated, and represented and by the various interests, institutions, and moral arguments that mobilized these efforts and resources." It is important to note, however, that Young strongly believes that PTSD is real. "The reality of PTSD is confirmed empirically by its place in people's lives, by their experiences and convictions, and by the personal and collective investments that have been made in it." Allan Young, *The Harmony of Illusions: Inventing Post-Traumatic Stress Disorder* (Princeton, NJ, 1995), p. 5. The vast literature on shell shock in Britain cannot be delineated here, but for one of the most recent works, see Peter Leese, *Shell Shock: Traumatic Neurosis and the British Soldiers of the First World War* (New York, 2002).
4. Jay Winter, "Shell-Shock and the Cultural History of the Great War," *Journal of Contemporary History*, 35, 1 (2000), 7–11, 7, 8.
5. See Adrian Gregory, *The Silence of Memory: Armistice Day, 1919–1946* (Oxford, 1994); Thomas W. Laqueur, "Memory and Naming in the Great War," in John R. Gillis, ed., *Commemorations: The Politics of National Identity* (Princeton, 1994); Jay Winter, *Sites of Memory, Sites of Mourning: The Great War in European Cultural History* (Cambridge, 1995); Jay Winter and Antoine Prost, *The Great War in History: Debates and Controversies, 1914 to the Present* (Cambridge, 2005); Joanna Bourke, *Dismembering the Male: Men's Bodies, Britain and the Great War* (London, 1996); Alison Light, *Forever England: Femininity, Literature and Conservatism Between the Wars* (London, 1991).
6. Billie Melman, "Introduction," in Melman, ed., *Borderlines: Genders and Identities in War and Peace, 1870–1930* (New York, 1998), p. 15.
7. See, among a large literature, Barbara Bush, *Imperialism, Race and Resistance: Africa and Britain, 1919–1945* (London, 1999); Laura Tabili, *"We Ask for British Justice," Workers and Racial Difference in Later Imperial Britain* (Ithaca, 1994); E.H. Green, *Ideologies of Conservatism: Conservative Political Ideas in the Twentieth Century* (Oxford, 2002); Joanna Alberti, *Beyond Suffrage: Feminists in War and Peace* (New York, 1989); Harold L. Smith, ed., *British Feminism in the Twentieth Century* (Aldershot, 1990); Tony Kushner and Kenneth Lund, eds,

Traditions of Intolerance: Historical Perspectives on Fascism and Race Discourse in Britain (Manchester, 1989); Barbara Storm Farr, *The Development and Impact of Ridht-Wing-Politics in Britain, 1903–1932* (1987); Mike Cronin, ed., *The Failure of British Fascism: The Far Right and the Fight for Political Recognition* (London, 1996); Julie V. Gottlieb, *Feminine Fascism: Women in Britain's Fascist Movement, 1923–1945* (London, 2000); Julie V. Gottlieb and Thomas P. Linehan, eds, *The Culture of Fascism: Visions of the Far Right in Britain* (London, 2004); Gillian Peele and Chris Cook, eds, *The Politics of Reappraisal, 1918–1939* (New York, 1975); John Turner, *British Politics and the Great War, Coalition and Conflict, 1915–1918* (New Haven, 1992); Philip Williamson, *National Crisis and National Government: British Politics, the Economy and Empire, 1926–1932* (Cambridge, 1992); Maurice Cowling, *The Impact of Labour, 1920–1924: The Beginning of Modern British Politics* (London, 1971); Kenneth O. Morgan, *Consensus and Disunity: The Lloyd George Coalition Government, 1918–1922* (Oxford, 1979); Ross McKibbin, *The Ideologies of Class: Social Relations in Britain, 1880–1950* (Oxford, 1994).

8. David Jarvis, "The Shaping of Conservative Electoral Hegemony, 1918–1939," in Jon Lawrence and Miles Taylor, eds, *Party, State and Society: Electoral Behaviour in Britain since 1920* (Aldershot, 1997), pp. 134, 146–147.

9. Susan Pedersen, "From National Crisis to 'National Crisis:' British Politics, 1914–1931," *Journal of British Studies*, 33 (3 July 1994), 322–335. See Jon Lawrence's well-argued "Forging a Peaceable Kingdom: War, Violence, and Fear of Brutalization in Post-First World War Britain," *Journal of Modern History*, 75 (September 2003), 557–589, for one of the conspicuous exceptions.

10. See Renato Rosaldo, "Grief and a Headhunter's Rage: On the Cultural Force of Emotions," in Edward M. Bruner, ed., *Text, Play, and Story: The Construction and Reconstruction of Self and Society* (Washington, D.C., 1984).

11. Bob Bushaway, "Name Upon Name: The Great War and Remembrance," in Roy Porter, ed., *Myths of the English* (Cambridge, 1992), p. 161. See also Helen McCarthy, "Parties, Voluntary Associations, and Democratic Politics in Interwar Britain," *The Historical Journal*, 50, 4 (2007), 891–912.

12. Philip Williamson, "The Doctrinal Politics of Stanley Baldwin," in Michael Bentley, ed., *Public and Private Doctrine: Essays in British History presented to Maurice Cowling* (Cambridge, 1993), pp. 184, 185, 188, 189, 191, 195.

13. Maurice Cowling, *The Impact of Labour, 1920–1924: The Beginning of Modern British Politics* (London, 1971), p. 70.

14. Eric L Santner, *Stranded Objects: Mourning, Memory, and Film in Postwar Germany* (Ithaca, NY, 1990), pp. 32, 33.

15. Jenny Edkins, "Remembering Relationality: Trauma Time and Politics," in Duncan Bell, ed., *Memory, Trauma and World Politics: Reflections on the Relationship Between Past and Present* (London, 2006), p. 110.

16. Hal Foster, "Armour Fou," *October*, 56 (Spring 1991), 95; "Postmodernism in Parallax,"*October*, 63 (Winter 1993), 10.

17. Janet K. Watson, *Fighting Different Wars: Experience, Memory, and the First World War in Britain* (New York, 2004), passim.

18. Edkins, "Remembering Relationality," pp. 104, 101, 108.

19. See letter from Leo Amery to Bonar Law, 24 October 1922, Amery Papers, AMEL 4 October 1922. My thanks to Jon Lawrence for making this available to me.

20. Peter Mandler, *The English National Character: The History of an Idea from Edmund Burke to Tony Blair* (New Haven, 2006), pp. 150, 143, 145, 147.
21. Dan Stone, *Breeding Superman: Nietzsche, Race and Eugenics in Edwardian and Interwar Britain* (Liverpool, 2002), Introduction.

1 Britons' Shattered Psyche

1. Samuel Hynes, *A War Imagined: The First World War and British Culture* (New York, 1992).
2. Jean Comaroff, "Aristotle Re-membered," in James Chandler, Arnold I. Davidson, and Harry Harootunian, eds, *Questions of Evidence: Proof, Practice, and Persuasion across the Disciplines* (Chicago, 1991), pp. 463–469; Quoted in Wolfgang Schivelbusch, *The Railway Journey: The Industrialization of Time and Space in the 19th Century* (Berkeley, 1986; originally published 1977), p. 164.
3. Quoted in Jonathan Rose, *The Edwardian Temperament, 1895–1919* (Athens, OH, 1986), pp. 199, 200, 201, 202.
4. Judith Lewis Herman, *Trauma and Recovery: The Aftermath of Violence—From Domestic Abuse to Political Terror* (New York, 1992), pp. 1, 1–2, 38, 51–56; Dori Laub, "Truth and Testimony: The Process and the Struggle," in Cathy Caruth, ed., *Trauma: Explorations in Memory* (Baltimore, 1995), p. 67.
5. Quoted in Judd, *Ford Madox Ford*, pp. 295–296; A Corporal, *Field Ambulance Sketches* (London, 1919), pp. 85, 95, 96, 20, 21; quoted from Laurence Housman, ed., *War Letters of Fallen Englishmen* (London, 1930), pp. 216, 62, 75.
6. In Housman, ed., *War Letters of Fallen Englishmen*, pp. 193, 296, 298, 300, 91, 193, 162–163, 164; quoted in Judd, *Ford Madox Ford*, p. 289.
7. Frederic Manning, *Her Privates We* (London, 1986), p. 196. Originally published as *The Middle Parts of Fortune* in 1929; Richard Aldington, *Death of a Hero* (New York, 1929), pp. 385, 355; Guy Chapman, *A Passionate Prodigality: Fragments of Autobiography* (New York, 1966, first published 1933), pp. 267, 269.
8. Jay Winter, *The Great War and the British People* (Cambridge, Ma., 1986), pp. 71–72.
9. Adrian Gregory, *The Silence of Memory: Armistice Day, 1919–1946* (Oxford, 1994), p. 19.
10. Phillip Gibbs, *The Hope of Europe* (London, 1921), pp. 287–288. Quoted in Hilary Spurling, *Ivy, The Life of I. Compton-Burnett* (New York, 1984), p. 229.
11. Caroline Playne, *A Society at War* (Boston, 1931), p. 131.
12. Gregory, *Silence of Memory*, p. 52.
13. Cited in Martin Stone, "Shellshock and the Psychologists," in W.F. Bynum, Roy Porter, and Michael Shepherd, eds, *The Anatomy of Madness: Essays in the History of Psychiatry, Volume II: Institutions and Society* (London, 1985), p. 249; Jay Winter, *The Great War and the British People* (London, 1986), p. 84.
14. E. Sylvia Pankhurst, *The Home Front: A Mirror to Life in England During the First World War* (London, 1987, first published 1932), p. 115; Trevor Wilson, *The Myriad Faces of War: Britain and the Great War, 1914–1918* (Cambridge, 1986), p. 157; Mrs. A. Burnett Smith [Annie S. Swan], *An Englishwoman's Home* (New York, 1918). pp. 23, 24, 29, 48. See the account in Susan R. Grayzel, *Women's*

Identities at War. Gender, Motherhood, and Politics in Britain and France during the First World War (Chapel Hill, NC, 1999).

15. Wilson, *Myriad Faces*, p. 509.
16. Siegfried Sassoon, *Memoirs of an Infantry Officer* (New York, 1930), p. 284; Playne, *Society*, p. 142; Gibbs, *Hope of Europe*, p. 288.
17. Introduction to Irene Rathbone, *We That Were Young* (New York, 1989, first published 1932), pp. x, xii; WAAC, *The Woman's Story of the War* (London, 1930), p. 195.
18. Angela Woollacott, *On Her Their Lives Depend: Munitions Workers in the Great War* (Berkeley, 1994), pp. 80, 84; Quoted in Gail Braybon and Penny Summerfield, *Out of the Cage: Women's Experiences in Two World Wars* (London, 1987), p. 85.
19. Storm Jameson, *Journey From the North: Autobiography of Storm Jameson*, Vol. I (London, 1969), p. 102, 104; quoted in Hilary Spurling, *Ivy, The Life of I. Compton-Burnett* (New York, 1984), pp. 238, 244; Burnett Smith, *An Englishwoman's Home*, pp. 19, 109; quoted in Tate, *Modernism*, pp. 10, 15; Vera Brittain, quoted in Spurling, *Ivy*, p. 229.
20. Playne, *Society*, p. 130.
21. Mary Dexter, *In the Soldier's Service: War Experiences of Mary Dexter* (Boston, 1918), pp. 108–109, 116.
22. Great Britain, Ministry of Health, *Report on the Pandemic of Influenza, 1918–1919* (London, 1920–1921), pp. iv, xiv, 69.
23. Ministry of Health, *Pandemic*, p. 67; "The Prevention of Influenza," *The Lancet* (1 March 1919), p. 347.
24. "Growing Toll of Influenza," *Daily Express* (3 July 1918), p. 3; Charles Graves, *Invasion By Virus: Can It Happen Again?* (London, 1969), p. 32; *Illustrated London News* (20 July 1918), p. 83; *Daily Express* (31 October 1918), p. 3; *Daily Express* (15 October 1918), p. 3; David Thomson and Robert Thomson, *Influenza*. Annals of the Pickett-Thomson Research Laboratory, Monograph XVI, Part I (London, 1933), p. 738; *British Medical Journal* (5 April 1919), p. 418.
25. *The Lancet* (26 October 1918), letter from William Collier, p. 567; Eileen Pettigrew, *The Silent Enemy: Canada and the Deadly Flu of 1918* (Saskatoon, 1983), p. 16; Ministry of Health, *Pandemic*, p. 72.
26. Caroline E. Playne, *Britain Holds On, 1917, 1918* (London, 1933), p. 389; *British Medical Journal* (17 August 1918), p. 159; *The Lancet* (1 February 1919), p. 196; quoted in Graves, *Invasion by Virus*, pp. 25–26; Thomson and Thomson, *Influenza*, pp. 789, 796; Sir Thomas Horder, M.D., "Some Observations on the More Severe Cases of Influenza Occurring During the Present Epidemic," *The Lancet* (28 December 1918), p. 872.
27. Spurling, *Ivy*, pp. 238, 239.
28. Katherine Anne Porter, "Pale Horse, Pale Rider," *The Collected Stories of Katherine Anne Porter* (New York, 1965), p. 309, 309–310.
29. Anthony Burgess, *Little Wilson and Big God* (London, 1987), pp. 17–20, 87–88.
30. Herman, *Trauma and Recovery*, p. 57; Kai Erikson, "Notes on Trauma and Community," in Cathy Caruth, ed., *Trauma: Explorations in Memory* (Baltimore, 1995), pp. 185, 194. Italics in the original; Cathy Caruth, "Introduction to Part I," in Caruth, ed., *Trauma*, p. 4; Herman, *Trauma and Recovery*,

p. 2. While some theorists deny that the dynamics of collective trauma can be understood in the same ways as those that characterize individual trauma, Jenny Edkins, taking a Lacanian position, argues that the distinctions between the individual and the social are false ones. Rather, the individual subject and the society in which he or she lives are "mutually constituted, neither one coming before the other but both being produced together" through language. As a consequence, she asserts, "trauma can never be a purely individual event, in the same way as there cannot be a private language, because it always already involves the community or the cultural setting in which people are placed. Imbricated in the social order, subjects operate within a contested arena of language that is only partial and incomplete, where meaning shifts and slides and cannot be tied resolutely to any single or final object;" this situation ensures that "answers to the awkward questions about life, death, survival" cannot be satisfactorily given. The questions themselves, in consequence, are rendered invisible or are forgotten altogether through the mobilization of what Lacan calls a "master signifier," a term or concept that serves as the organizing principle of the social order to which all other meanings attach themselves, thereby stabilizing meaning and enabling subjects to make sense of the society or culture within which they live. Such master signifiers include God, the Nation, Communism, the Jew, Woman—concepts, we shall see, that appear regularly in the political struggles that take place in 1920s Britain. See Jenny Edkins, "Remembering Relationality: Trauma Time and Politics,", pp. 103, 104, 101, 106, 108.

31. Larry R. Squire and Eric R. Kandel, *Memory from Mind to Molecules* (New York, 1999), pp. 213, 6; quoted in Bessel A. Van der Kolk and Onno Van der Hart, "The Intrusive Past: The Flexibility of Memory and the Engraving of Trauma," in Cathy Caruth, ed., *Trauma: Explorations in Memory* (Baltimore, 1995), pp. 169, 170; Jeffrey C. Alexander, "Toward a Theory of Cultural Trauma," in Jeffrey C. Alexander, Ron Eyerman, Bernhard Giesen, Neil J. Smelser, and Piotr Sztompka, eds, *Cultural Trauma and Collective Identity* (Berkeley, 2004), p. 22.

32. Charles R. Figley and Rolf J. Kleber, "Beyond the 'Victim:' Secondary Traumatic Stress," in Rolf J. Kleber, Charles R. Figley, D. Berthold P.R. Gersons, *Beyond Trauma: Cultural and Societal Dynamics* (New York, 1995), pp. 78, 93.

33. Tate, *Modernism*, p. 10.

34. Rebecca West, *The Return of the Soldier* (New York, 1980; originally published 1918), p. 137; Dorothy L. Sayers, "The Unsolved Puzzle of the Man with No Face," in Dorothy L. Sayers, ed., *Lord Peter Views the Body* (New York, 1986), p. 216; Dorothy L. Sayers, *Unnatural Death* (New York, 1987; originally published 1927), pp. ix, x.

35. Elizabeth von Arnim, *The Enchanted April* (London, 1922), pp. 153, 155–156, 201; Rose Macaulay, *What Not, A Prophetic Comedy* (London, 1919), pp. x, 1.

36. See Carolyn J. Dean, *The Self and Its Pleasures: Bataille, Lacan, and the History of the Decentered Subject* (Ithaca, 1992), pp. 5, 15, 50–51.

37. Hal Foster, "Postmodernism in Parallax," *October*, 63 (Winter 1993), 3–20, 8; quoted in Larry Ray, "Mourning, Melancholia and violence," in Bell., ed., *Memory, Trauma and World Politics: Reflections on the Relationship Between Past and Present* (London, 2006), p. 145.

38. Judd, *Ford Madox Ford*, p. 320; Subaltern, *Subaltern's War*, p. 190; C.E. Montague, *Disenchantment* (New York, 1922), p. 255; Rathbone, *We That Were Young*, p. 449.
39. Subaltern, *Subaltern's War*, p. 205; Graves, *Goodbye to All That* (New York, 1957; originally published 1929), pp. 287, 268, 293; Judd, *Ford Madox Ford*, p. 320.
40. J.R. Ackerley, *My Father and Myself* (New York, 1968), p. 216; Geoffrey Moorhouse, *Hell's Foundations: A Social History of the Town of Bury in the Aftermath of the Gallipoli Campaign* (New York, 1992), p. 109; Vera Brittain, *Testament of Youth* (London, 1978; originally published 1933), p. 496.
41. Rathbone, *We That Were Young*, pp. 422–423; Ackerley, *My Father and Myself*, p. 217; Moorhouse, *Hell's Foundations*, pp. 107–108, 198–199.
42. Herbert Read, *The Contrary Experience* (London, 1973; originally published 1963), pp. 66, 67; Chapman, *Passionate Prodigality*, pp. 276, 280, 281.
43. Gregory, *Silence of Memory*, p. 54.
44. Rathbone, *We That Were Young*, p. 430; Richard Aldington, *Life for Life's Sake* (London, 1941), p. 189, 188, 187; Subaltern, *Subaltern's War*, p. 208; Carrington, *A Subaltern's War*, p. 259; Philip Gibbs, *Now It Can Be Told* (New York, 1920), pp. 551–552.
45. Richard Aldington, *Death of a Hero*, p. 308; Robert Graves, *Good-bye To All That*, p. 321, Subaltern, *Subaltern's War*, p. 253; Judd, *Ford Madox Ford*, p. 323; Paul Fussell, *The Great War and Modern Memory* (New York, 1975), passim, Vera Brittain, *Testament of Experience* (New York, 1957); *Testament of Friendship* (London, 1940); *Testament of Youth*.
46. Quoted in Gregory, *Silence of Memory*, pp. 9, 11; Laqueur, "Memory and Naming in the Great War," pp. 158, 161; Bushaway, "Name Upon Name,"; Gregory, *Silence of Memory*, pp. 4, 5; Ray, "Mourning, Melancholia and Violence," pp. 145, 151, 136.
47. Herman, *Trauma and Recovery*, pp. 214, 70; As Hal Foster has argued, the answers to what he calls "the quintessential modern question"—who are we?—have been arrived at "by way of an appeal to an otherness, either to the unconscious within or to cultural others without." Foster, "Postmodernism," p. 8.

2   Jews, "Blacks," and the Promises of Radical Conservatism, 1919–1925

1. F.D. Lugard, "The Colour Problem," *The Edinburgh Review*, pp. 233, 466 (April 1921), pp. 267–283, 269.
2. Philip Gibbs, *Now It Can Be Told*, pp. 547–548.
3. This and the following three paragraphs are drawn from Susan Kingsley Kent, *Making Peace: The Reconstruction of Gender in Interwar Britain* (Princeton, 1993), Ch. 5.
4. See Jarvis, "The Shaping of Conservative Electoral Hegemony"; Morgan, *Consensus and Disunity*; Cowling, *The Impact of Labour*; Green, *Ideologies of Conservatism*.
5. Quoted in Kent, *Making Peace*, Ch. 2.

6. Rathbone, *We That Were Young*, pp. 431–432.

7. Lady Rhondda, *This Was My World* (London, 1933), p. 294.

8. Kent, *Making Peace*.

9. Billie Melman, ed., *Borderlines: Genders and Identities in War and Peace, 1870–1930* (New York, 1998), pp. 15, 17–18.

10. Quoted in Panikos Panayi, *The Enemy in Our Midst: Germans in Britain During the First World War* (New York, 1991), pp. 96, 221.

11. Ann Dummett and Andrew Nicol, *Subjects, Citizens, Aliens and Others: Nationality and Immigration Law* (London, 1990), p. 107.

12. House of Commons, *Debates* (15 April 1919), col. 2765; "The Undesirable Bill," *Daily Mail* (16 April 1919), p. 6.

13. Kenneth O. Morgan, *Consensus and Disunity*, pp. 238–239; Dummett and Nicol, *Subjects, Citizens, Aliens and Others*, p. 112.

14. House of Commons, *Debates* (15 April 1919), cols. 2763, 2779, 2791, 2792.

15. Ibid., cols. 2798, 2797, 2801; 23 October 1919, col. 189.

16. House of Commons, *Debates* (23 October 1919), cols. 198, 209–210.

17. House of Commons, *Debates* (15 April 1919), cols. 2784, 2792; House of Commons, *Debates* (22 October 1919), col. 65.

18. House of Commons, *Debates* (15 April 1919), col. 2784; "The Superior Attitude," *Morning Post* (20 December 1919), p. 6; House of Commons, *Debates* (22 October 1919), col. 76; House of Commons, *Debates* (15 April 1919), cols. 2787, 2778; House of Commons, *Debates* (22 October 1919), col. 86.

19. House of Commons, *Debates* (15 April 1919), col. 2778.

20. House of Commons, *Debates* (18 November 1919), col. 839; House of Commons, *Debates* (15 April 1919), cols. 2763, 2772, 2784; House of Commons, *Debates* (22 October 1919), col. 88; House of Commons, *Debates* (13 November 1919), col. 542; House of Commons, *Debates* (22 October 1919), col. 103.

21. House of Commons, *Debates* (2 May 1905), col. 710; House of Commons, *Debates* (18 April 1905), col. 465, 467; House of Commons, *Debates* (5 August 1914), col. 1989.

22. Tony Kushner, "The Paradox of Prejudice: The Impact of Organised Anti-semitism in Britain during an Anti-Nazi War", in Tony Kushner and Kenneth Lunn, eds, *Traditions of Intolerance: Historical Perspectives on Fascism and Race Discourse in Britain* (Manchester, 1989), p. 79.

23. Panikos Panayi, "Introduction," in Panayi, ed., *Racial Violence in Britain, 1840–1950* (Leicester, 1993), p. 11. Some scholars will take issue with the interpretation offered here, seeing the riots more in class terms than I have acknowledged here. See Laura Tabili, *"We Ask for British Justice:" Workers and Racial Difference in Late Imperial Britain* (Ithaca, 1994); Jon Lawrence, "Forging a Peaceable Kingdom: War, Violence, and Fear of Brutalization in Post-First World War Britain," *Journal of Modern History*, 75 (September 2003), 557–589.

24. Tabili, *"We Ask for British Justice,"* pp. 17, 135.

25. Jacqueline Jenkinson, "The 1919 Race Riots in Britain: Their Background and Consequences," unpublished thesis (University of Edinburgh, 1987), pp. 55, 56, 58.

26. Jenkinson, "The 1919 Race Riots in Britain," p. 91.

27. Quoted in Jenkinson, "The 1919 Race Riots in Britain," pp. 109, 114.

28. Ibid., "The 1919 Race Riots in Britain," pp. 172, 174, 175.
29. Jenkinson, "The 1919 Race Riots in Britain," p. 245.
30. Quoted in Jenkinson, "The 1919 Race Riots in Britain," p. 221.
31. See Lawrence, "Forging a Peaceable Kingdom," p. 567.
32. "Negro Hunt by a Wild Cardiff Crowd," *South Wales Evening Express and Evening Mail* (13 June 1919). Front page; quoted in Jenkinson, "The 1919 Race Riots in Britain," p. 159; "Race Riots: The Root Cause," *Daily Herald* (13 June 1919), p. 4.
33. *South Wales Evening Express and Evening Mail* (12 June 1919). Front Page, Quoted in Jenkinson, "The 1919 Race Riots in Britain," p. 160; "The Colour Problem," *Cardiff Times and South Wales Weekly News* (5 July 1919), p. 8; " 'We Are Loyal,' " *Cardiff Times and South Wales Weekly News* (21 June 1919), p. 8.
34. *South Wales Evening Express and Evening Mail* (13 June 1919). Front Page, "Negro Hunt by a Wild Cardiff Crowd."
35. "Race Riots: The Root Cause," *The Daily Herald* (13 June 1919), p. 4; "Battles Renewed in Cardiff," *The Daily Herald* (14 June 1919), p. 4.
36. "Black and White at Liverpool," *The Times* (10 June 1919), p. 9; *The Times* (14 June 1919), p. 8. "East-End Racial Feud," *Daily Chronicle* (17 June 1919), p. 3; "Race Rioting at Cardiff," *The Times* (13 June 1919), p. 9.
37. Paul B. Rich, *Race and Empire in British Politics* (Cambridge, 1986), p. 117; "The Negro Riots. A Lesson for England." *Morning Post* (13 June 1919), p. 12; quoted in Jenkinson, "The 1919 Race Riots in Britain," p. 177.
38. Quoted in Jenkinson, "The 1919 Race Riots in Britain," p. 159.
39. Ibid., pp. 187, 188, 192; Jon Lawrence, personal communication.
40. Quoted in Jenkinson, "The 1919 Race Riots in Britain," pp. 186–187.
41. Tabili, *"We Ask for British Justice,"* p. 121.
42. Barbara Bush, *Imperialism, Race and Resistance: Africa and Britain, 1919–1945* (London, 1999), p. 209.
43. Robert Reinders, "Racialism on the Left. E.D. Morel and the 'Black Horror on the Rhine," *International Review of Social History*, 13 (1968), pp. 1–28, 8, 5.
44. *Daily Herald* (9 April 1920), front page.
45. "Outrage on Womanhood," *Daily Herald* (10 April 1920), front page.
46. "A NEW HORROR," *Daily Herald* (10 April 1920), p. 4. Italics in the original.
47. *Daily Herald* (4 April 1920), p. 4; 13 April 1920, front page.
48. E.D. Morel, *The Horror on the Rhine* (London, April 1921), pp. 10, 13. Italics in the original.
49. E.D. Morel, "Black Troops in Germany. The Use of non-European Peoples by European governments for European Wars and for the Prosecution of Political and Diplomatic Ends in Europe," *Special Supplement to 'Foreign Affairs,'* (June 1920), v–x. (Verbatim report of a speech at the meeting held at the Central Hall, Westminster, on 27 April [1920], organized by the Women's International League, Mrs. H.M. Swanwick in the chair.), ix.
50. W.H. Dawson, "Germany and Spa," *Contemporary Review*, CXVIII (July 1920), pp. 1–12, 8.
51. *The Nation* (10 April 1920), p. 29; "A London Diary," by A Wayfarer, Ibid., p. 37.
52. "Our French Alliance," *Woman's Leader* (16 April 1920), p. 240; "Black Troops Again," (13 August 1920), p. 616.
53. Thomas Jones, *Diary*, 1 (8 April 1920), p. 108.

54. F.D. Lugard, "The Colour Problem," *The Edinburgh Review*, pp. 233, 466 (April 1921), pp. 267–283, 267, 268, 280, 283, 269.
55. Barbara Ehrenreich, Introduction to Klaus Theweleit, *Male Fantasies, Volume I: Women, Floods, Bodies, History* (Minneapolis, 1987, original 1977), p. xiv; Theweleit, Vol. II, pp. 3, 76. My italics; Theweleit, Vol. II, pp. 74, 75.
56. Quoted in Kushner and Lunn, "Introduction," in Kushner and Lunn eds, *Traditions of Intolerance*, p. 2; Kenneth Lunn, "The Ideology and Impact of the British Fascists in the 1920s," in Kushner, Tony and Kenneth Lund, eds, *Traditions of Intolerance: Historical Perspectives on Fascism and Race Discourse in Britain* (Manchester, 1989), p. 152; Kushner and Lunn, *Traditions of Intolerance*, pp. 6, 3.
57. Kenneth Lunn, "The Ideology and Impact of the British Fascists in the 1920s," pp. 146–147.
58. David Baker, "The Extreme Right in the 1920s: Fascism in a Cold Climate or 'Conservatism with the Knobs On'"? in Mike Cronin, ed., *The Failure of British Fascism: The Far Right and the Fight for Political Recognition* (London, 1996), p. 17.
59. G.C. Webber, *The Ideology of the British Right, 1918–1939* (London, 1986), p. 28.
60. "The Cause of World Unrest," *Morning Post* (21 July 1920), p. 7; "The Cause of World Unrest," *Morning Post* (27 July 1920), p. 7; "The Bolshevist Plot in England," *Morning Post* (4 August 1920), p. 5; "The Greatest Peril," *Morning Post* (17 July 1920), p. 6.
61. Webber, *The Ideology of the British Right*, p. 57.
62. "A Home Office Problem," *The Times* (27 November 1924), p. 18; "Alien London," (28 November 1924), p. 15; "Alien London," (4 December 1924), p. 15; "Alien London," (8 December 1924), pp. 15–16.
63. David Cesarani, "Joynson-Hicks and the Radical Right in England After the First World War," in Kushner and Lunns, eds, *Traditions of Intolerance: Historical Perspectives on Fascism and Race Discourse in Britain* (Manchester, 1989), p. 128.
64. Bryan Cheyette, "Jewish Stereotyping and English Literature, 1875–1920: Towards a Political Analysis," in Kushner and Lunn, eds, *Traditions of Intolerance: Historical Perspectives on Fascism and Race Discourse in Britain* (Manchester, 1989), p. 29.
65. Quoted in Cesarani, "Joynson-Hicks and the Radical Right," p. 129; the quote is from *The Times* (13 December 1924). In Hansard, "refuse" was changed to "regiment." Fn. 56, p. 137
66. Ross McKibbin, *The Ideologies of Class: Social Relations in Britain, 1880–1950* (Oxford, 1994), p. 275; Caesarani, "Joynson-Hicks and the Radical Right," p. 134; Harriette Flory, "William Joynson-Hicks, Lord Brentford: A Political Biography," unpublished dissertation (University of Cincinnati, 1975); G.C. Webber, *The Ideology of the British Right, 1918–1939* (New York, 1986), pp. 28, 18, 2. J. Stevenson, "Conservatism and the Future of Fascism in Interwar Britain," in M. Blinkhorn, ed., *Fascists and Conservatives* (London, 1990), pp. 275–276.
67. Webber, *Ideology of the British Right*, pp. 55, 56, 57.

3 The Amritsar Massacre, 1919–1920

1. Quoted in Nigel Collett, *The Butcher of Amritsar: General Reginald Dyer* (London, 2005), pp. 270, 205.
2. Quoted in Derek Sayer, "British Reaction to the Amritsar Massacre, 1919–1920," *Past and Present*, 131 (1991), pp. 130–164, 160.
3. Collett, *Butcher of Amritsar*, p. 223.
4. Meston, "Quo Vadis in India," *The Contemporary Review*, CXVIII (October 1920), pp. 457–465, 458; *The Times* (16 April 1919), p. 12.
5. Collett, *Butcher of Amritsar*, p. 227.
6. Government of India, *Disorders Inquiry Report, 1919–1920, Volume II* (Calcutta, 1920), pp. 32, 33.
7. Quoted in Collett, *Butcher of Amritsar*, p. 237.
8. Collett, *Butcher of Amritsar*, p. 241.
9. House of Lords, *Debate*, "Punjab Disturbances: The Case of General Dyer," (19–20 July 1920), col. 262; Collett, *Butcher of Amritsar*, pp. 248–249.
10. Quoted in Rupert Furneaux, *Massacre at Amritsar* (London, 1963), p. 75.
11. Quoted in Collett, *Butcher of Amritsar*, p. 55.
12. Collett, *Butcher of Amritsar,* p. 257.
13. Montagu letter prefacing report of *Disorders Inquiry Committee, 1919–1920, Report* (Calcutta, 1920), pp. xliv; 44.
14. *Disorders Inquiry Committee Report*, pp. 47, 188, 191, 195.
15. Report of the Commissioners Appointed by the Punjab Sub-Committee of the Indian National Congress, 1920 (New Delhi, 1976 reprint), pp. 56–57.
16. Quoted in Collett, *Butcher of Amritsar*, p. 270.
17. *Disorders Inquiry Committee Report*, p. 204.
18. Quoted in Collett, *Butcher of Amritsar*, pp. 284, 281, 285.
19. Derek Sayer, "British Reaction to the Amritsar Massacre, 1919–1920," *Past and Present*, p. 131 (May 1991), 130–164, 152.
20. Quoted in Collett, *Butcher of Amritsar*, pp. 212, 211, 205, 261, 264.
21. *Disorders Inquiry Committee Report*, p. xliv; Collett, *Butcher of Amritsar*, pp. 423, 357.
22. House of Lords, *Debate*, "Punjab Disturbances: The Case of General Dyer," (19–20 July 1920), col. 260.
23. *Morning Post* (18 December 1919), p. 6; An Englishwoman, "Amritsar," *Blackwood's Magazine*, CCVII (April 1920), pp. 441–446, 442, 443, 444–445; Ian Colvin, *The Life of General Dyer* (London, 1929), pp. 145, 143, 146, 178; House of Commons, *Debate* on "Punjab Disturbances. Lord Hunter's Committee," (8 July 1920), cols. 1705–1820, 1714; House of Lords, *Debate*, "Punjab Disturbances: The Case of General Dyer," (19–20 July 1920), col. 373.
24. Ian Colvin, *The Life of General Dyer*, p. 177; *Morning Post* (18 December 1919), p. 6; *Morning Post* (15 December 1919), p. 9; House of Lords, *Debate*, "Punjab Disturbances: The Case of General Dyer," (19–20 July 1920), cols. 229, 296, 252; *Spectator* (3 January 1920).
25. House of Commons, *Debate* on "Punjab Disturbances. Lord Hunter's Committee," (8 July 1920), cols. 1705–1820, 1735; House of Lords, *Debate*, "Punjab Disturbances: The Case of General Dyer," (19–20 July 1920), col.

228; "What Happened at Amritsar," *Morning Post* (15 December 1919), p. 9.

26. House of Lords, *Debate*, "Punjab Disturbances: The Case of General Dyer," (19–20 July 1920), cols. 297, 225; "The Well and the Garden," *Morning Post* (18 December 1919), p. 6; "The Amritsar Shooting," *Morning Post* (30 December 1919), p. 4; An Englishwoman, "Amritsar," 446.

27. *Morning Post* (15 December 1919), p. 9; *Morning Post* (6 July 1920), p. 7; "The European in India," *Morning Post* (6 July 1920), p. 6.

28. Collett, *Butcher of Amritsar*, p. 225 ; quoted in Furneaux, *Massacre at Amritsar*, pp. 93, 94, 95; quoted in Collett, *Butcher of Amritsar*, p. 284.

29. Quoted in Collett, *Butcher of Amritsar*, p. 367; House of Lords, *Debate*, "Punjab Disturbances: The Case of General Dyer," (19–20 July 1920), cols. 230, 341–342.

30. Quoted in Collett, *Butcher of Amritsar*, pp. 364, 367; "Dyer Saved India," *Morning Post* (7 July 1920), p. 8. Italics in the original.

31. Quoted in Collett, *Butcher of Amritsar*, p. 349; "Burning Questions: Two opinions on Amritsar.'Sipahi,' " "English Women and Amritsar," *Women's Leader* (27 August 1920), pp. 658–659.

32. These quotes come from *The Times* (17 September 1857, 29 August 1857, 5 June 1858, 17 December 1857, 17 September 1857).

33. House of Lords, *Debate*, "Punjab Disturbances: The Case of General Dyer," (19–20 July 1920), cols. 222–378.

34. House of Commons, *Debate* on "Punjab Disturbances. Lord Hunter's Committee," (8 July 1920), cols. 1705–1820, 1708, 1710; House of Lords, *Debate*, "Punjab Disturbances: The Case of General Dyer," (19–20 July 1920), cols. 222–378, 284; House of Commons, *Debate* on "Punjab Disturbances. Lord Hunter's Committee," (8 July 1920), cols. 1705–1820, 1777, 1739.

35. "To Redress A Wrong," *Morning Post* (16 July 1920), p. 6; Commons, *Debate* on "Punjab Disturbances. Lord Hunter's Committee," (8 July 1920), cols. 1705–1820, 1712, 1719; House of Lords, *Debate*, "Punjab Disturbances: The Case of General Dyer," (19–20 July 1920), cols. 258, 289; *Morning Post* (10 July 1920), p. 6.

36. House of Commons, *Debate* on "Punjab Disturbances. Lord Hunter's Committee," (8 July 1920), cols. 1778, 1795, 1803; "To Redress a Wrong," *Morning Post* (16 July 1920), p. 6.

37. Quoted in Collett, *Butcher of Amritsar*, pp. 379–380, 380, 381.

38. *Morning Post* (10 July 1920), p. 6; Sayers, "British Reaction to the Amritsar Massacre, 1919–1920," p. 157.

39. *Morning Post* (14 July 1920), p. 7, fund appeal; quoted in Sayers, "British Reaction to the Amritsar Massacre, 1919–1920," p. 157; quoted in Collett, *Butcher of Amritsar*, p. 388.

40. *Disorders Inquiry Committee Report*, p. 194.

41. House of Commons, *Debate* on "Punjab Disturbances. Lord Hunter's Committee," (8 July 1920), cols. 1707, 1728, 1728–1729, 1730, 1746.

42. House of Lords, *Debate*, "Punjab Disturbances: The Case of General Dyer," (19–20 July 1920), cols. 350, 353, 366, 300, 304, 274; "Dyer Case. Vindication of Important Principle." *Daily Chronicle* (9 July 1920), p. 4.

43. House of Commons, *Debate* on "Punjab Disturbances. Lord Hunter's Committee," (8 July 1920), cols. 1725, 1727–1778, 1736, 1739.

44. House of Lords, *Debate*, "Punjab Disturbances: The Case of General Dyer," (19–20 July 1920), col. 296, House of Commons, *Debate* on "Punjab Disturbances. Lord Hunter's Committee," (8 July 1920), col. 1778; House of Lords, *Debate*, "Punjab Disturbances: The Case of General Dyer," (19–20 July 1920), cols. 373, 373–375; Sayer, "British Reaction to the Amritsar Massacre, 1919–1920," pp. 135, 153; *Morning Post* (20 July 1920), pp. 4, 6, coverage of Lords debate on Dyer next to reports of "Irish Anarchy," p. 4; *Morning Post* (10 July 1920), p. 7, part of Dyer fund appeal.

45. House of Lords, *Debate*, "Punjab Disturbances: The Case of General Dyer," (19–20 July 1920), cols. 279, 263.

46. "The Peril of the Military Mind," *The Nation* (20 December 1919), p. 413.

47. Quoted in Sayer, "British Reaction to the Amritsar Massacre, 1919–1920," p. 153; Manchester *Guardian* (9 July 1920) editorial.

4 Reprisals in Ireland, 1919–1921

1. General Neville Macready to Sir John Anderson, marked SECRET, no date, but either 26 or 27 September 1920. Henry Wilson papers (HHW) 2/2B/9.

2. Charles Gore, letter to *The Times* (19 November 1920), p. 6.

3. Charles Townshend, *Political Violence in Ireland: Government and Resistance since 1848* (Oxford, 1983), pp. 299, 302, 306.

4. Quoted in Townshend, *Political Violence*, p. 308.

5. D.G. Boyce, *Englishmen and Irish Troubles: British Public Opinion and the Making of Irish Policy, 1918–1922* (London, 1972), p. 43.

6. Quoted in Townshend, *Political Violence*, p. 332.

7. "Formation of a Special Force for Service in Ireland," from Churchill, as Sec'y of War, to Cabinet (19 May 1920). PRO WO 32/9517; Boyce, *Englishmen and Irish Troubles*, pp. 50, 85; David Neligan, *The Spy in the Castle* (London, 1999, first published 1968), p. 173.

8. Thomas Jones, *Whitehall Diary, Volume III: Ireland, 1918–1925* (London, 1971), p. xxi; Tim Pat Coogan, *Michael Collins: The Man Who Made Ireland* (Boulder, CO, 1996; originally published 1992), p. 124; see Dorothy Macardle, *The Irish Republic, A Documented Chronicle of the Anglo-Irish Conflict and the Partitioning of Ireland, with a Detailed Account of the Period 1916–1923* (Dublin, 1999; originally published 1937), pp. 429, 433, 461n, 730, 801.

9. Irish Situation, 1920. Situation in Ireland Committee, Cabinet. PRO CAB 27/108.

10. Jones, *Whitehall Diary, Volume III*, p. 53; "Report on the situation in Ireland" (29 June 1920); Greenwood report to SIC (26 July 1920), p. 80; Greenwood to SIC (13 September 1920), pp. 172, 172–173, 184–185; Coogan, *Michael Collins*, p. 145; Greenwood to SIC, for week ending (23 December 1920).

11. Douglas V. Duff, *Sword for Hire: The Saga of a Modern Free-Companion* (London, 1934), pp. 65, 61, 62, 65–66, 75–76.

12. Duff, *Sword for Hire*, pp. 87, 88, 89–90.

13. Quoted in Coogan, *Michael Collins*, pp. 165, 125, 126; House of Lords Record Office, Papers of Andrew Bonar Law.

14. "More Irish Reprisals," *The Times* (28 September 1920), p. 10; Hugh Martin, *Ireland in Insurrection: An Englishman's Record of Fact* (London, 1921), p. 120.

15. Daniel J. Murphy, ed., *Lady Gregory's Journals, Volume I* (New York, 1978), pp. 199, 205, 192.
16. See House of Commons, *Debate* (21 February 1921), col. 627; Murphy, ed., *Gregory Journal*, pp. 189, 196, 196–197, 276.
17. Murphy, ed., *Gregory Journal*, pp. 208, 209, 209–210; Coogan, *Michael Collins*, pp. 145–146.
18. Martin Gilbert, *Churchill, A Life* (New York, 1991), pp. 422–423; Macready/ Wilson letters from IWM; 11/11/20, HHW 2/2C/1; Jones, *Diary*, p. 53; Duff, *Sword for Hire*, p. 77; "Up the Rebels," *Weekly Summary* (4 March 1921), p. 1.
19. Michael Hopkinson, ed., *The Last Days of Dublin Castle: The Diaries of Mark Sturgis* (Dublin, 1999), pp. 27, 49; Gilbert, *Churchill*, p. 425; Sturgis, *Diaries*, p. 52; Coogan, *Michael Collins*, p. 156.
20. Winston S. Churchill, *The World Crisis, 1918–1928: The Aftermath* (New York, 1929), p. 298; Gilbert, *Churchill*, p. 426; A History of the 5th Division in Ireland (November 1919–March 1922). Typescript, n.d. Papers of Lieutenant-General Sir Hugh Jeudwine, Imperial War Museum, Box 78/82/2, p. 44.
21. *Weekly Summary* (8 October 1920), p. 4; (4 March 1921), p. 1; (24 June 1921), p. 1.
22. Sturgis, *Diaries*, p. 25; Macready to Wilson (1 September 1920).
23. Macready to Wilson (28 August 1920); (24 September 1920); M to Anderson, marked SECRET, no date, but either 26 or 27 September 1920, HHW 2/2B/9; Macready to Wilson (25 September 1920); (28 September 1920).
24. Macready to Wilson (22 September 1920); (7 October 1920); Churchill, *Aftermath*, p. 302; Macready to Wilson (14 October 1920).
25. Wilson to Macready (13 October 1920, 14 October 1920); Letter from Lloyd George to Sir Hamar Greenwood, Chief Secretary for Ireland, dated (25 February 1921). House of Lords Record Office, Papers of David Lloyd George, F/19/3/4.
26. Jones, *Diary*, p. 33; Macready to Wilson (25 September 1920, 26 September 1920).
27. Keith Jeffery, ed., *The Military Correspondence of Field Marshal Sir Henry Wilson, 1918–1922* (London, 1985), p. 266.
28. The Irish Situation Committee, Record of Meetings, 1920–1921. PRO CAB 27/107. Minutes of ISC meeting 16th June 1921.
29. Macready to Anderson, marked SECRET, no date, but either 26 or 27 September 1920, HHW 2/2B/9; Churchill, *Aftermath*, p. 49; Gibbs, *Hope of Europe*, pp. 221, 221–222.
30. General Headquarters, the Forces in Ireland, "Record of the Rebellion in Ireland in 1920–21 and the Part Played by the Army in Dealing with It." Vol. II: Intelligence. Papers of Lieutenant-General Sir Hugh Jeudwine, Imperial War Museum, Box 78/82/2, 1922, p. 31; Jon Lawrence, "Forging a Peaceable Kingdom: War, Violence, and Fear of Brutalization in Post-First World War Britain," pp. 557–589, 580; Gregory, *Diary* (16 December 1920), pp. 213–214; Duff, *Sword for Hire*, pp. 19, 25.
31. Duff, *Sword for Hire*, pp. 26, 26–27, 29, 30, 32, 33.
32. Ibid., pp. 33, 34, 41; Herman, *Trauma and Recovery*, p. 44.
33. A History of the 5th Division in Ireland (November 1919–March 1922). Typescript, n.d. Papers of Lieutenant-General Sir Hugh Jeudwine, Imperial War Museum, Box 78/82/2, p. 64; General Headquarters, the Forces in Ireland,

"Record of the Rebellion in Ireland in 1920–21 and the Part Played by the Army in Dealing with It." Vol. I: Operations, Papers of Lieutenant-General Sir Hugh Jeudwine, Imperial War Museum, Box 78/82/2, 1922, p. 33. A History of the 5th Division in Ireland (November 1919–March 1922). Typescript, n.d. Papers of Lieutenant-General Sir Hugh Jeudwine, Imperial War Museum, Box 78/82/2, p. 50; *Weekly Summary* (27 May 1921), p. 4. Appendix A, "Some Notes on the Duties of Intelligence Officers," (18 July 1921), by J. Brind, of the General Staff, General Headquarters, the Forces in Ireland, "Record of the Rebellion in Ireland in 1920–21 and the Part Played by the Army in Dealing with It." Vol. II: Intelligence. Papers of Lieutenant-General Sir Hugh Jeudwine, Imperial War Museum, Box 78/82/2, 1922, p. 54.

34. Appendix A, "Some Notes on the Duties of Intelligence Officers," (18 July 1921), by J. Brind, of the General Staff, General Headquarters, the Forces in Ireland, "Record of the Rebellion in Ireland in 1920–21 and the Part Played by the Army in Dealing with It." Vol. II: Intelligence. Papers of Lieutenant-General Sir Hugh Jeudwine, Imperial War Museum, Box 78/82/2, 1922, p. 54. General Headquarters, the Forces in Ireland, "Record of the Rebellion in Ireland in 1920–21 and the Part Played by the Army in Dealing with It." Vol. I: Operations, Papers of Lieutenant-General Sir Hugh Jeudwine, Imperial War Museum, Box 78/82/2, 1922, p. 33. A History of the 5th Division in Ireland (November 1919–March 1922). Typescript, n.d. Papers of Lieutenant-General Sir Hugh Jeudwine, Imperial War Museum, Box 78/82/2, pp. 64, 68, 73; Churchill, Gibbs here on shirking war; *Weekly Summary* of (3 June 1921), p. 1; Sturgis, *Diaries*, p. 4; Wilson to Macready (29 June 1920), HHW 2/2A/31; Martin, *Ireland in Insurrection*, p. 59.
35. *Weekly Standard* (15 April 1921); Sturgis, *Diaries*, pp. 93, 95.
36. Duff, *Sword for Hire*, pp. 34, 77.
37. Irish Situation Committee, Record of Meetings, 1920–1921. PRO CAB 27/107 (22 July 1920); General Headquarters, the Forces in Ireland, "Record of the Rebellion in Ireland in 1920–21 and the Part Played by the Army in Dealing with It." Vol. I: Operations, Papers of Lieutenant-General Sir Hugh Jeudwine, Imperial War Museum, Box 78/82/2, 1922, p. 34; Appendix XIV, p. 1. History of the 5th General Headquarters, the Forces in Ireland, "Record of the Rebellion in Ireland in 1920–21", pp. 140, 135, 142.
38. Boyce, *Englishmen and Irish Troubles*, pp. 50–51; "Mr. Asquith on Irish Reprisals," *The Times* (30 October 1920), p. 12; Gibbs, *Hope of Europe*, p. 219.
39. Gibbs, *Hope of Europe*, pp. 219, 220.
40. Boyce, *Englishmen and Irish Troubles*, p. 63; Gibbs, Foreward to Martin, *Ireland in Insurrection*, p. 11; *The Times* (1 November 1920), p. 13; *Intellectual Manifesto*—no date, no place of publication, but 1921; "Report of the British Labor [sic] Commission to Ireland," 1921, no date, no place of publication, p. 34.
41. Gibbs in Martin, *Insurrection in Ireland*, pp. 13–14; Gibbs, *Hope of Europe*, pp. 74, 75; General Headquarters, the Forces in Ireland, "Record of the Rebellion in Ireland in 1920–21 and the Part Played by the Army in Dealing with It." Vol. II: Intelligence. Papers of Lieutenant-General Sir Hugh Jeudwine, Imperial War Museum, Box 78/82/2, 1922, p. 32; Wilson, *Diaries* (18 May 1921); Churchill, *Aftermath*, p. 295.
42. Gibbs, *Hope of Europe*, pp. 74, 115, 115–116.

43. Irish Situation Committee, Record of Meetings, 1920–1921. PRO CAB 27/107. Draft Conclusions of 26 May 1921; Churchill, *Aftermath*, p. 315; Wilson, *Diaries*, Wilson to Milne (2 June 1920), pp. 177–178.
44. "Report of the British Labor [*sic*] Commission to Ireland," pp. 5, 6.
45. Macready to Wilson (1 November 1920).

5   The General Strike of 1926

1. *The Times* (6 May 1926), p. 3.
2. Hannon, House of Commons (3 May 1926), col. 147; Churchill called it a "shocking disaster in our national life" Churchill, House of Commons (3 May 1926), col. 116; quoted in Julian Symons, *The General Strike: A Historical Portrait* (London, 1957), p. 57; Anne Olivier Bell, ed., *The Diary of Virginia Woolf, Vol. III, 1925–1930* (New York, 1980), 5 May 1926, p. 77; Symons, *The General Strike*, p. 57; Woolf, *Diary*, p. 77.
3. Many sections of the British public did not accept this picture of the working classes, to the chagrin of conservatives who believed that the threat of labor was not taken seriously enough. My thanks to Jon Lawrence for this corrective.
4. Barbara Storm Farr, *The Development and Impact of Right-Wing Politics in Britain, 1903–1932* (1987), pp. 38, 39.
5. Farr, *Right-Wing Politics*, p. 39; Aldington, *Death of a Hero*, p. 206; Thomas Jones, *Whitehall Diary Volume I: 1916–1925* (London, 1969), 4 April 1921, pp. 134, 135, 136.
6. E.H.H. Green, *Ideologies of Conservatism*, pp. 120, 126–127, 128; Jones, *Diary*, p. 80.
7. McKibbin, *Ideologies of Class*, pp. 283, 284; Green, *Ideologies of Conservatism*, p. 134.
8. Quoted in Keith Middlemas and John Barnes, *Baldwin, A Biography* (London, 1969), p. 123.
9. McKibbin, *Ideologies of Class*, p. 287.
10. Quoted in Anne Perkins, *A Very British Strike: 3 May–12 May 1926* (London, 2006), p. 35; quoted in Flory, *William Joynson-Hicks*, p. 90; *The Times* (3 May 1924), p. 7; quoted in Lewis Chester, Stephan Fay, Hugo Young, *The Zinoviev Letter* (Philadelphia, 1968), p. 126.
11. Cesarani, in Kushner and Lunn, eds, *Traditions of Intolerance*, p. 128; quoted in Chester, et al., *Zinoviev Letter*, p. 127; Perkins, *Very British Strike*, p. 46.
12. "Class Hatred," *Daily Mail* (25 October 1924), p. 6.
13. "Moscow's Orders," *Daily Mail* (25 October 1924), p. 8.
14. "Vote Conservative," *Daily Mail* (29 October 1924), p. 8.
15. "Under Which Flag?", *Daily Mail* (29 October 1924), p. 9.
16. *Daily Mail* (31 October 1924), pp. 9, 8.
17. Quoted in Perkin, *Very British Strike*, p. 49.
18. Quoted in Flory, *William Joynson-Hicks*, p. 124; quoted in Perkins, *Very British Strike*, p. 73; "Subversive Propaganda" (21 April 1926). House of Commons, *Debates*, cols. 1301, 1302, 1310, 1312, 1322.
19. Quoted in Farr, *Right-Wing Politics*, pp. 57, 58; quoted in Perkins, *Very British Strike*, p. 72.

20. Letter from Joynson-Hicks to Baldwin (1 September 1925), quoted in Richard Charles Maguire, " 'The Fascists . . . are . . . to be depended upon.' The British Government, Fascists and Strike-breaking during 1925 and 1926," in Nigel Copsey and David Renton, eds, *British Fascism, the Labour Movement and the State* (Basingstoke, 2005), p. 8; minute by A. Dixon (27 July 1925), quoted in Maguire, " 'The Fascists,' " p. 19; Cabinet meeting minutes (7 October 1925), quoted in Maguire, " 'The Fascists,' " p. 20.
21. "INDUSTRIAL CRISIS. FAILURE OF NEGOTIATIONS." House of Commons, *Debates* (3 May 1926), cols. 72, 73, 124–125.
22. See Samuel Hynes, *A War Imagined: The First World War and English Culture* (New York, 1991), ch. 20; "Speech before House, May 6, 1926," in Sir John Simon, *Three Speeches on the General Strike* (London, 1926), p. 2; Speech before House (11 May 1926), pp. 24–25, 29.
23. *The Times* (6 May 1926), pp. 3, 5.
24. "A Menace to the Nation," *The Times* (3 May 1926), p. 15; "The Voice of Parliament," (4 May 1926), p. 9.
25. *Daily Mail* (3 May 1926), p. 8; *Daily Mail*, strike edition, typescript, no date.
26. *Mayfair Bulletin* (4 May 1926); Perkins, *Very British Strike*, pp. 173, 174; *British Gazette* (8 May 1926); *Daily Express* (8 May 1926); Woolf, *Diaries*, Vol. 3 (12 May 1926), p. 85; quoted in Hynes, *A War Imagined*, p. 411.
27. "Battalion Arrives at Cardiff," *Daily Mail* (3 May 1926), p. 9 (6 May 1926, 10 May 1926, 11 May 1926); *British Gazette* (7 May 1926, 8 May 1926); *The Times* (8 May 1926), p. 8 (10 May 1926), p. 2.
28. Quoted in Perkin, *Very British Strike*, p. 140; Margaret Cole, ed., *Beatrice Webb's Diaries, 1914–1932* (London, 1956), p. 93; Perkin, *Very British Strike*, pp. 143, 180–181; *Daily Mail* (11 May 1926); quoted in Perkin, *Very British Strike*, p. 179; *British Gazette* (5 May 1926).
29. Quoted in Perkin, *Very British Strike*, p. 159; H. Duckworth, "Diary of General Strike," typescript, London School of Economics archives.
30. Quoted in Maguire, " 'Fascists,' " p. 18.
31. Perkin, *Very British Strike*, p. 217; "SUPPLY," House of Commons, *Debates* (10 May 1926), cols. 718, 718–719.
32. House of Commons, *Debates* (3 May 1926), col. 74; "Trustees for Nation," *Daily Herald* (19 April 1926), p. 2; "Will Mr. Baldwin Do His Duty?" *Daily Herald* (20 April 1926), p. 4; " 'A Crime Against Society,' " *Daily Herald* (3 May 1926), p. 4; "The Issue," *Daily Herald* (4 May 1926), p. 4; House of Commons, *Debates* (7 May 1926), col. 674; "Wonderful Response to the Call," *British Worker* (5 May 1926).
33. *British Worker* (5 May 1926); "Our Reply to 'Jix,' " *British Worker* (6 May 1926); "Loyal Obedience to TUC. Orders," *British Worker* (7 May 1926).
34. "Strikers Wear War Medals," *British Worker* (7 May 1926); "The Miners are *Not* 'Bluffing,' " *Daily Herald* (28 May 1926), p. 4; *Daily Herald* (19 May 1926), p. 4; House of Commons, *Debates* (10 May 1926), cols. 739–740, 742, 780.
35. *The Daily Herald* (19 May 1926), p. 4; Woolf, *Diaries* (13 May 1926), p. 85; Patrick Renshaw, *The General Strike* (London, 1975), p. 252.
36. Charles Loch Mowat, *Britain Between the Wars, 1918–1940* (Chicago, 1955), p. 337; quoted in *Public Opinion* (21 May 1926), p. 451.

37. C.F.G. Masterson, "The General Strike and After," *The Contemporary Review*, CXXIX (June 1926), 683, 687; Keith Laybourn, *The General Strike of 1926* (Manchester, 1993), p. 111; Renshaw, *General Strike*, pp. 242, 248.
38. To be sure, papers like the *Morning Post* and the *Daily Express* were making this case on the eve of the strike. I am grateful to Jon Lawrence for pointing this out to me.
39. "The Defeat of the General Strike. The Analogy of War," *The Nation and Atheneum*, XXXIV, 6 (15 May 1926), 158.
40. "For King and Country. Revolution Routed," *Daily Mail* (13 May 1926), p. 2; "England's Example," *Daily Mail* (14 May 1926), p. 2; "No Reprisals," *Daily Mail* (15 May 1926), p. 2.
41. "The Nation's Victory," *The Times* (13 May 1926), p. 3; "Reinstatement," *The Times* (14 May 1926), p. 3.
42. Masterson, "The General Strike and After," pp. 686–687; Simon, *Three Speeches*, pp. 55, 53.
43. *The Times* (14 May 1926), p. 3; "Life and Politics," *The Nation and Atheneum*, XXXIV, 7 (22 May 1926), pp. 169–170, 171, 172.
44. Simon, *Three Speeches*, pp. ix, xv, 46; quoted in *Public Opinion* (21 May 1926), p. 451.
45. *Daily Mail* (13 May 1926); Simon, *Three Speeches*, p. xiv; quoted in "The Progress of Modern Science and Mechanism Really Gained the Day," *Public Opinion* (21 May 1926), p. 451.
46. Stanley Baldwin, *Our Inheritance: Speeches and Addresses by the Right Honourable Stanley Baldwin, M.P* (London, 1928), pp. 224, 220, 221–222; Sir William Joynson-Hicks, *Communist Plotting: Lessons from the General Strike* (National Union of Conservative and Unionist Associations, 1926), p. 3.
47. "Life and Politics," *The Nation and Atheneum*, XXXIV (7, 22 May 1926), pp. 169, 170.

6 Flappers and the Igbo Women's War of 1929 (with Marc Matera)

1. Lt. Col. P.F. Pritchard, "More Deadly Than the Male," (Narrative rejected for publication April 1957), undated, Documents Collection, Imperial War Museum (74/121/1), p. 4.
2. Testimony before the *Aba Commission of Inquiry: Notes of Evidence* (August 1930), The Royal Empire Society, Received 11 March 1931, pp. 114–115, paragraph 2321.
3. "Talks with Woman," *Daily Mail* (28 October 1924), p. 6; "Do Our Statesmen Understand," *Daily Mail* (31 October 1924), p. 8.
4. See Susan Kingsley Kent, *Making Peace*, Ch.5.
5. Quoted in Susan Kingsley Kent, *Gender and Power in Britain, 1640–1990* (London, 1999), Ch. 12.
6. Billie Melman, *Women and the Popular Imagination in the Twenties: Flappers and Nymphs* (New York, 1988), p. 1.
7. Quoted in Melman, *Women and Popular Imagination*, pp. 18–19.
8. *Daily Mail* (22 November 1927), p. 11; quoted in Melman, *Women and Popular Imagination*, pp. 19–20.

9. See Susan Kingsley Kent, *Making Peace.*
10. Quoted in Melman, *Women and Popular Imagination*, p. 20.
11. *Daily Mail* (11 April 1927), p. 11; (14 April 1927), p. 10; "Why Not Drop It?" (16 April 1927), p. 8; (12 April 1927), p. 9; (25 April 1927), p. 10.
12. (26 April 1927), p. 10. "Stop the Flapper-Vote Folly," *Daily Mail* (11 April 1927), p. 10; "Flapper Vote Folly," *Daily Mail* (26 April 1927), p. 11. "Why Socialists Want Votes for 'Flappers.'" *Daily Mail* (20 April 1927), p. 10. (23 April 1927), p. 9. *Daily Mail* (8 December 1927), p. 15. *Daily Mail* (8 December 1927), p. 15. *Daily Mail* (8 December 1927), p. 15. *Daily Mail* (31 August 1928), p. 11.
13. *Daily Mail* (28 April 1927), p. 10; (23 November 1927), p. 10; (30 July 1928), p. 11; (14 December 1927), p. 15; (13 December 1927), p. 15; (20 December 1927), p. 8.
14. *Daily Mail* (6 December 1927), p. 7; *Daily Mail* (12 May 1928), p. 12; (3 June 1929), p. 10; (5 June 1929), p. 11.
15. *Daily Express* (13 April 1927), pp. 1, 8; (15 April 1927), p. 9; (25 April 1927), pp. 3, 8.
16. House of Commons, Representation of the People (Equal Franchise) Bill (29 March 1928), col. 1431; quoted in *Daily Mail* (22 November 1927), p. 11; House of Commons, Representation of the People (Equal Franchise) Bill (29 March 1928), cols. 1359, 1360, 1366, 1367.
17. House of Commons, Representation of the People (Equal Franchise) Bill (29 March 1928), cols. 1443, 1379, 1380, 1381, 1383, 1388–1389.
18. Ibid., cols. 1398, 1400, 1401, 1434.
19. Ibid., cols. 1454, 1456, 1457, 1459.
20. See Susan Kingsley Kent, *Sex and Suffrage in Britain, 1860–1914* (Princeton, 1987); and Kent, *Making Peace.*
21. House of Commons, Representation of the People (Equal Franchise) Bill (29 March 1928), cols. 1473, 1474, 1476, 1476–1477.
22. Ibid., cols. 1388, 1390, 1407, 1409.
23. Adrian Bingham, *Gender, Modernity, and the Popular Press in Inter-War Britain* (Oxford, 2004), p. 201.
24. *The Times* (30 May 1928), p. 16; The *Guardian* (30 March 1928), p. 10; "The Flapper Vote," *The Times* (22 May 1929), p. 14; "Incidents of the Poll," The *Guardian* (31 May 1920), p. 13; *Times* (19 April 1928), p. 16; *Times* (6 May 1929), p. 11; The *Guardian* (1 May 1929), p. 11; (2 May 1929), p. 8; Letter to the Editor by Ernest J.P. Benn, *Times* (21 May 1929), p. 19; *Times* (1 May 1929), p. 13; (2 May 1929), p. 9; (22 May 1929), p. 8; The *Guardian* (30 May 1929), p. 10.
25. *Times* (28 May 1929), p. 8; *Times* (30 May 1929), p. 8; *Guardian* (30 May 1929), pp. 11, 12; *Guardian* (31 May 1929), p. 13; *Times* (29 May 1929), p. 9.
26. The *Guardian* (20 May 1929), p. 20; *The Times* (1 May 1929), p. 6; *Guardian* (1 May 1929), p. 11; *The Times* (2 May 1929), p. 9; *Guardian* (2 May 1929), p. 9, (3 May 1929), p. 13, (10 May 1929), p. 17; *Guardian* (15 May 1929), p. 7, *Guardian* (18 May 1929), p. 18; *Times* (20 May 1929), p. 10; *Guardian* (30 May), p. 12.
27. *Times* (31 May 1929), p. 12; *Guardian* (1 June 1929), p. 18.
28. *Daily Mail* (1 May 1929), p. 9; "Watering Down the Franchise," *Daily Mail* (13 December 1927), p. 15; *National Review* (14 November 1927), p. 10; *Daily*

Mail (29 August 1928), p. 11; *Daily Mail* (15 June 1928), p. 6, (16 June 1928), p. 11; see, for example, *Daily Mail* (19 December 1927), p. 6; (9 December 1927), p. 8; "Can Conservativism Be Saved?" *Daily Mail* (10 June 1929), p. 10; Gregory, *Silence of Memory*, p. 119.

29. See Misty Bastian, " 'Vultures of the Marketplace': Igbo and Other Southeastern Nigerian Women's Discourse about the Ògù Umùnwaànyi (Women's War) of 1929," in Jean Allman, Susan Geiger and Nakanyike Musisi, eds, *Women and African Colonial History* (Bloomington, 2001).

30. See Judith Van Allen, " 'Sitting On a Man:' Colonization and the Lost Political Institutions of Igbo Women," in Sharon W. Tiffany, ed., *Women and Society: An Anthropological Reader* (St. Albans, VT, 1979).

31. Colonial Office, *Minutes of Evidence Taken by a Commission of Inquiry Appointed to Inquire into Certain Incidents at Opobo, Abak and Utu Etim Ekpo in December, 1929*, by Major William Birrell Gray, chairman, January 1930, in *Aba Commission of Inquiry: Notes of Evidence*, Annexure II, Appendix III (14) (a), The Royal Empire Society, Received 11 March 1931, p. 31.

32. Lt. Col. P.F. Pritchard, "More Deadly Than the Male" (Narrative rejected for publication April 1957), undated, Documents Collection, Imperial War Museum (74/121/1), London SE1, p. 4.

33. See Bush, *Imperialism, Race and Resistance*, p. 88.

34. Margaret Green, *Igbo Village Affairs* (London, 1964), pp. 201, 202, 203, 205.

35. T. Obinkaram Echewa, *I Saw the Sky Catch Fire* (New York, 1992), pp. 145–146.

36. Colonial Office, *Minutes of Evidence Taken by a Commission of Inquiry Appointed to Inquire into Certain Incidents at Opobo, Abak and Utu Etim Ekpo in December, 1929*, by Major William Birrell Gray, chairman, January 1930, in *Aba Commission of Inquiry: Notes of Evidence*, Annexure II, Appendix III (14) (a), The Royal Empire Society, Received 11 March 1931, p. 7.

37. United Kingdom, Public Record Office (CO 169/2), "Report by Mr. A.R. Whitman, D.O.," confidential dispatch received 6 January 1930, nos 93 (p. 8, paragraph 56 of report).

38. United Kingdom, Public Record Office (CO 583/169/2), "An Inquisition Taken at Opobo," by coroner for the Opobo Division, taken and sworn before S.T. Harvey, 24 December 1929, nos 153.

39. United Kingdom, Public Record Office (CO 583/169/3), "An Inquisition Taken at Utu Etim Ekpo on 26 December 1929, by Karl Vernon Hanitsch, Coroner of the Ikot Ekpene Division," nos 47–48.

40. Public Record Office (CO 583/169/3), "An Inquisition Taken at Utu Etim Ekpo on 26 December 1929, by Karl Vernon Hanitsch, Coroner of the Ikot Ekpene Division," nos 53.

41. See Harry A. Gailey, *The Road to Aba: A Study of British Administrative Policy in Eastern Nigeria* (New York, 1970).

42. Governor Graeme Thomson telegram to Secretary of State Passfield, 3 February 1930, CO 583/169/14, p. 2; CO 583/168/14, no date, but appears to be 24 or 25 December 1929.

43. *The Times* (13 December 1929), p. 14.

44. *The Times* (16 December 1929), p, 12; (19 December 1929), pp. 13, 11; *Daily Mail* (19 December 1929), p. 5; (20 December 1929), p. 13.

45. *The Times* (24 December 1929), p. 11; (29 December 1929), p. 7; *Daily Mail* (28 December 1929), p. 10.

46. "The Disturbances in Nigeria. Inquiry Commission Appointed," *The Times* (31 January 1930), p. 14.

47. See "Nigerian Massacres," *Daily Worker* (4 January 1930), p. 5; and "Pacification by Rifles," *Daily Worker* (1 January 1930), p. 5.

48. Extract of 18 December 1929, in CO 583/168/14, item 7.

49. *The African World* (11 January 1930), p. 533; (18 January 1930), p. 583.

50. *The Spectator* (24 May 1930), p. 859.

51. "The Riots in Nigeria. A Revolt of Women," *The Times* (25 August 1930), p. 12.

52. "The Rioting in Nigeria," *Morning Post* (26 August 1930).

53. "Massacre of 54 Unarmed Women," *Daily Worker* (27 August 1930), p. 3.

54. House of Commons, *Parliamentary Debates* (5th Series), Vol. 233, cols 1392–1393, 1946–1947, 2155; Vol. 234, cols 1013–1015; Vol. 238, cols 951–952, 2408–2409; Vol. 239, cols 410–411.

55. House of Commons, *Parliamentary Debates* (12 November 1930), col. 1656.

56. See "Despatch from the Secretary of State for the Colonies to the officer Administering the Government of Nigeria regarding the Report of the Commission of Inquiry into the Distrubances at Aba and other places in South-Eastern Nigeria in November and December, 1929," Great Britain, Command Paper 3784, 1931, p. 4; and *Parliamentary Debates* (18 February 1931), cols. 1229–1230.

57. "Despatch from the Secretary of State," p. 4; CO 583/176/9, p. 62; C.T. Lawrence, Sec'y of Southern Provinces of Nigeria, to Chief Secretary to the Government in Lagos, 24 December 1929, CO 583/169/2.

58. *Aba Commission of Inquiry: Notes of Evidence*, p. 379, paragraph 7138.

59. Ibid., pp. 114–115, paragraph 2321.

60. Foster, "Postmodernism in Parallax," p. 10.

61. Ray, in Duncan, *Memory*, p. 139.

62. Neil J. Smelser, "Psychological Trauma and Cultural Trauma," in Alexander, et al., *Cultural Trauma and Collective Identity* (Berkeley, 2004), p. 53.

Conclusion: Resolving the "National Crisis" of 1929–1931

1. J.L. Garvin, editorial, "Patriotism as a Power. Class-War as Suicide." *The Observer* (13 September 1931), p. 14.

2. Margaret Cole, ed., *Beatrice Webb's Diaries, 1914–1932*, p. 294.

3. Philip Williamson, *National Crisis and National Government: British Politics, the Economy and Empire, 1926–1932* (Cambridge, 1992), p. 1. This chapter follows the argument made by Susan Pedersen in her important review essay, "From National Crisis to 'National Crisis': British Politics, 1914–1931," *Journal of British Studies*, 33, 3 (July 1994), 322–335, in which she criticizes Williamson for failing to place the political concerns of the 1929–1931 crisis in the context of the struggles over economy and politics in the immediate postwar years. I share her view that the disorders and crises of the postwar decade are of a piece, offering emotional, cultural, and psychological explanations for the social, financial, and political upheavals Pedersen identifies.

4. Mowat, *Britain Between the War*, p. 377.
5. Quoted in Williamson, *National Crisis*, pp. 1, 135.
6. "The Aftermath," *Daily Mail* (4 August 1931), p. 8.
7. Williamson, *National Crisis*, pp. 136, 153.
8. "The Nation and the Axe," *The Observer* (2 August 1931), p. 8.
9. Mowat, *Britain Between the Wars*, p. 393.
10. Cole, ed., *Beatrice Webb's Diaries*, p. 283.
11. Williamson, *National Crisis*, pp. 364, 365, 367.
12. Ibid., p. 388
13. Ibid., p. 344.
14. Quoted in Williamson, *National Crisis*, pp. 432, 427.
15. Ibid., p. 453.
16. *The Observer* (23 August 1931), p. 11: "Crisis and Deadlock"; J.L. Garvin, "Britain Yet?...The Coming Elections and Class-War. A Life-and-Death Fight." *The Observer* (30 August 1931), p. 10; "National Government-Limited," *The Observer* (30 August 1931), p. 10; J.L. Garvin, "Britain Yet?... The Coming Elections and Class-War. A Life-and-Death Fight." *The Observer* (30 August 1931), p. 10.
17. J.L. Garvin, "Britain Yet?...The Coming Elections and Class-War. A Life-and-Death Fight." *The Observer* (30 August 1931), p. 10; "'The War Over Again.'" *The Observer* (30 August 1931), p. 11; J.L. Garvin, "Britain Arise! Class or Country? Patriotism and Mass-Bribery," *The Observer* (6 September 1931), p. 12.
18. "Patriotism as a Power. Class-War as Suicide." *The Observer* (13 September 1931), p. 14; "The Eve of Battle." *The Observer* (4 October 1931), p. 16.
19. "Over the Top" *The Observer* (11 October 1931), p. 16; "Fighting to Win" *The Observer* (18 October 1931), p. 16; "The Day!" *The Observer* (25 October 1931), p. 14.
20. Winston S. Churchill, "The Way Out of the Crisis," *Daily Mail* (2 October 1931), p. 8; "A Warning to M.P.s," *The Daily Express* (27 August 1931), p. 8; "Now We Can See," *Daily Express* (7 October 1931), p. 10; "Next Tuesday Night," *Daily Express* (22 October 1931), p. 8.
21. Sir Philip Gibbs, "Is England Worth Saving?" *Daily Express* (26 October 1931), p. 8; "The Churches and the Election. A Call to Prayer. Duty of Christian People," *The Times* (15 October 1931), p. 16; "To Save England," *Daily Mail* (26 October 1931), p. 10; "Vote To-Day to Save the Nation and Yourself," *Daily Mail* (27 October 1931), p. 11; "The Call of Duty." *Daily Mail* (27 October 1931), p. 10.
22. "Not a National Government!" *Daily Herald* (25 August 1931), p. 8; "On Being British," *Daily Herald* (28 August 1931), p. 8.
23. "Who is the 'Nation'?" *Daily Herald* (5 October 1931), p. 8; "Unity for Victory" *Daily Herald* (6 October 1931), p. 8; "Tory Fist in the 'National' Glove" *Daily Herald* (9 October 1931), p. 8.
24. "More Cats Out of the Bag," *Daily Herald* (26 October 1931), p. 8.
25. Williamson, *National Crisis*, pp. 480, 455.
26. Ibid., p. 456.
27. Cole, ed., *Beatrice Webb's Diaries*, p. 294.
28. "The Stricken Field." *The Observer* (1 November 1931), p. 16.

29. "The Electoral Massacre of ex-Ministers." *The Observer* (1 November 1931), p. 16; *Daily Express* (28 October 1931), *Daily Mail* (28 October 1931), p. 9; "A Victory for Common Sense," *Daily Mail* (29 October 1931), p. 10.
30. Quoted in Williamson, *National Crisis*, pp. 458, 480, 455.
31. "WELL DONE!" *Daily Express* (28 October 1931), p. 8; "A Mighty Deed." *The Observer* (1 November 1931), p. 16.
32. As recounted by Stanley Baldwin, Cabinet minutes (27 November 1936), CAB 23/86, p. 7.
33. Kingsley Martin, *The Magic of Monarchy* (New York, 1937), p. 14.
34. "Constitutional Crisis. Attitude of the British Press," PREM 1/446.
35. *The Observer* (1 November 1931), p. 16: "A Mighty Deed."

Bibliography

Archive sources

Churchill College, Cambridge:
AMEL 4/10. Leo Amery Papers, 1922.
House of Lords Record Office:
Papers of Andrew Bonar Law.
Papers of David Lloyd George, F/19/3/4.
Imperial War Museum:
Henry Wilson papers (HHW) 2/2B/9.
Papers of Lieutenant-General Sir Hugh Jeudwine, Imperial War Museum, Box 78/82/2.
Pritchard, Lt. Col. P.F. "More Deadly Than the Male," undated, Documents Collection, 74/121/1.
London School of Economics:
Duckworth, H., "Diary of General Strike," undated.
Public Record Office:
CAB 23/86. Cabinet minutes, 27 November 1936.
CAB 27/101, 27/107, 27/108. Situation in Ireland Committee, 1920–1921.
CO 583/169/2. C.T. Lawrence, Sec'y of Southern Provinces of Nigeria, to Chief Secretary to the Government in Lagos, 24 December 1929.
CO 583/169/2. *"An Inquisition Taken at Opobo," by coroner for the Opobo Division, taken and sworn before S.T. Harvey, 24 December 1929.*
CO 583/169/2. *"Report by Mr. A.R. Whitman, D.O.," confidential dispatch received 6 January 1930.*
CO 583/169/3. "An Inquisition Taken at Utu Etim Ekpo on 26 December 1929, by Karl Vernon Hanitsch, Coroner of the Ikot Ekpene Division," 1929.
CO 583/169/14. "Minutes of Evidence Taken by a Commission of Inquiry Appointed to Inquire into Certain Incidents at Opobo, Abak and Utu Etim Ekpo in December, 1929".
PREM 1/446. "Constitutional Crisis. Attitude of the British Press," n.d.
WO 32/9517. "Formation of a Special Force for Service in Ireland," 1920.

Government documents

Great Britain, "Despatch from the Secretary of State for the Colonies to the officer Administering the Government of Nigeria regarding the Report of the Commission of Inquiry into the Disturbances at Aba and other places in South-Eastern Nigeria in November and December, 1929," Command Paper 3784, 1931.
Great Britain, Ministry of Health, *Report on the Pandemic of Influenza, 1918–1919.* London, 1920–1921.
Government of India, *Disorders Inquiry Report, 1919–1920, Volume II.* Calcutta: 1920.

House of Commons, *Parliamentary Debates*.
House of Lords, *Parliamentary Debates*.

Periodicals and newspapers

The African World
Blackwood's Magazine
British Gazette
British Medical Journal
British Worker
Cardiff Times and South Wales Weekly News
Contemporary Review
Daily Chronicle
Daily Express
Daily Herald
Daily Mail
Daily Worker
Guardian
Illustrated London News
Lancet
Mayfair Bulletin
Morning Post
The Nation
The Nation and Athenaeum
National Review
The Observer
Public Opinion
South Wales Evening Express and Evening Mail
Spectator
The Times
Weekly Summary
Woman's Leader

Primary sources

A Corporal, *Field Ambulance Sketches*. London, 1919.
Ackerley, J.R., *My Father and Myself*. New York, 1968.
Aldington, Richard, *Death of a Hero*. New York, 1929.
Aldington, Richard, *Life for Life's Sake*. London, 1941.
Baldwin, Stanley, *Our Inheritance: Speeches and Addresses by the Right Honourable Stanley Baldwin, M.P.* London, 1928.
Bell, Anne Olivier, ed., *The Diary of Virginia Woolf, Vol. III, 1925–1930*. New York, 1980.
Brittain, Vera, *Testament of Youth*. London, 1978; originally published 1933.
——, *Testament of Experience*. New York, 1957.
——, *Testament of Friendship*. London, 1940.
Burgess, Anthony, *Little Wilson and Big God*. London, 1987.
Burnett Smith, A. [Annie S. Swan], *An Englishwoman's Home*. New York, 1918.

Chapman, Guy, *A Passionate Prodigality: Fragments of Autobiography*. New York, 1966.

Chester, Lewis, Stephan Fay, and Hugo Young, *The Zinoviev Letter*. Philadelphia, 1968.

Churchill, Winston S., *The World Crisis, 1918–1928: The Aftermath*. New York, 1929.

Cole, Margaret, ed., *Beatrice Webb's Diaries, 1914–1932*. London, 1956.

Colvin, Ian, *The Life of General Dyer*. London, 1929.

Dawson, W.H., "Germany and Spa," *Contemporary Review*, CXVIII (July 1920), 1–12.

Dexter, Mary, *In the Soldier's Service: War Experiences of Mary Dexter*. Boston, 1918.

Duff, Douglas V., *Sword for Hire: The Saga of a Modern Free-Companion*. London, 1934.

Edmunds, Charles [pseudonym of Charles E. Carrington], *A Subaltern's War*. New York, 1930.

Ford, Ford Madox, *Parade's End*. New York, 1979.

Gibbs, Philip, *Heirs Apparent*. New York, 1924.

——, *The Hope of Europe*. London, 1921.

——, *Now It Can Be Told*. New York, 1920.

Graves, Robert, *Goodbye to All That*. New York, 1960; originally published 1929.

Green, Margaret, *Igbo Village Affairs*. London, 1964.

Hopkinson, Michael, ed., *The Last Days of Dublin Castle: The Diaries of Mark Sturgis*. Dublin, 1999.

Housman, Lawrence, ed., *War Letters of Fallen Englishmen*. London, 1930.

Jameson, Storm, *Journey From the North: Autobiography of Storm Jameson*, Vol. I. London, 1969.

Jeffery, Keith, ed., *The Military Correspondence of Field Marshal Sir Henry Wilson, 1918–1922*. London, 1985.

Lugard, F.D., "The Colour Problem," *The Edinburgh Review*, 233, 466 (April 1921), 267–283.

Rose, Macaulay, *What Not, A Prophetic Comedy*. London, 1919.

Manning, Frederic, *Her Privates We*. London, 1986.

Martin, Hugh, *Ireland in Insurrection: An Englishman's Record of Fact*. London, 1921.

Martin, Kingsley, *The Magic of Monarchy*. New York, 1937.

Masterson, C.F.G., "The General Strike and After," *The Contemporary Review*, CXXIX (June 1926).

Maxwell, W.N., *A Psychological Retrospect of the Great War*. London, 1923.

Meston, "Quo Vadis in India," *The Contemporary Review CXVIII* (October 1920), 457–465.

Middlemas, Keith, ed., *Thomas Jones, Whitehall Diary*. London, 1969.

Montague, C.E., *Disenchantment*. New York, 1922.

Morel, E.D., "Black Troops in Germany. The Use of non-European Peoples by European governments for European Wars and for the Prosecution of Political and Diplomatic Ends in Europe," *Special Supplement to 'Foreign Affairs,'* (June 1920), v–xi.

——, *The Horror on the Rhine*. London, 1921.

Murphy, Daniel, J., ed., *Lady Gregory's Journals, Volume I*. New York, 1978.

Pankhurst, E. Sylvia, *The Home Front: A Mirror to Life in England During the First World War*. London, 1987; originally published 1932.

Pettigrew, Eileen, *The Silent Enemy: Canada and the Deadly Flu of 1918*. Saskatoon, 1983.
Playne, Caroline, E., *Britain Holds On, 1917, 1918*. London, 1933.
——, *Society at War, 1914–1916*. Boston, 1931.
Porter, Katherine Anne, "Pale Horse, Pale Rider," *The Collected Stories of Katherine Anne Porter*. New York, 1965.
Rathbone, Irene, *We That Were Young*. New York, 1989, first published 1932.
Read, Herbert, *The Contrary Experience*. London, 1973; originally published 1963.
Report of the British Labor [sic] Commission to Ireland, 1921.
Report of the Commissioners Appointed by the Punjab Sub-Committee of the Indian National Congress. 1920. New Delhi, 1976; reprint.
Rhondda, *This Was My World*. London, 1933.
Sassoon, Siegfried, *Memoirs of an Infantry Office*. New York, 1930.
Sayers, Dorothy, L., *Unnatural Death*. New York, 1987.
——, "The Unsolved Puzzle of the Man with No Face," in Dorothy L. Sayers, ed., *Lord Peter Views the Body*. New York, 1986.
Simon, Sir John, *Three Speeches on the General Strike*. London, 1926.
Thomson, David and Robert Thomson, *Influenza*. Annals of the Pickett-Thomson Research Laboratory, Monograph XVI, Part I. London, 1933.
Von Arnim, Elizabeth, *The Enchanted April*. London, 1922.
WAAC, *The Woman's Story of the War*. London, 1930.
West, Rebecca, *The Return of the Soldier*. New York, 1980; originally published 1918.

Secondary sources

Alberti, Joanna, *Beyond Suffrage: Feminists in War and Peace*. New York, 1989.
Baker, David, "The Extreme Right in the 1920s: Fascism in a Cold Climate or 'Conservatism with the Knobs On'"? in Mike Cronin, ed., *The Failure of British Fascism: The Far Right and the Fight for Political Recognition*. London, 1996.
Bastian, Misty, " 'Vultures of the Marketplace': Igbo and Other Southeastern Nigerian Women's Discourse about the Ògù Umùnwaànyi (Women's War) of 1929," in Jean Allman, Susan Geiger and Nakanyike Musisi, eds, *Women and African Colonial History*. Bloomington, 2001.
Bingham, Adrian, *Gender, Modernity, and the Popular Press in Inter-War Britain*. Oxford, 2004.
Bourke, Joanna, *Dismembering the Male: Men's Bodies, Britain and the Great War*. London, 1996.
Boyce, D.G., *Englishmen and Irish Troubles: British Public Opinion and the Making of Irish Policy, 1918–1922*. London, 1972.
Braybon, Gail and Penny Summerfield, *Out of the Cage: Women's Experiences in Two World Wars*. London, 1987.
Bush, Barbara, *Imperialism, Race and Resistance: Africa and Britain, 1919–1945*. London, 1999.
Bushaway, Bob, "Name Upon Name: The Great War and Remembrance," in Roy Porter, ed., *Myths of the English*. Cambridge, 1992.
Cesarani, David, "Joynson-Hicks and the Radical Right in England After the First World War," in Kushner, Tony and Kenneth Lund, eds, *Traditions of*

Intolerance: Historical Perspectives on Fascism and Race Discourse in Britain. Manchester, 1989.

Cheyette, Bryan, "Jewish Stereotyping and English Literature, 1875–1920: Towards a Political Analysis," in Kushner, Tony and Kenneth Lund, eds, *Traditions of Intolerance: Historical Perspectives on Fascism and Race Discourse in Britain.* Manchester, 1989.

Collett, Nigel, *The Butcher of Amritsar: General Reginald Dyer.* London, 2005.

Comaroff, Jean, "Aristotle Re-membered," in James Chandler, Arnold I. Davidson, and Harry Harootunian, eds, *Questions of Evidence: Proof, Practice, and Persuasion across the Disciplines.* Chicago, 1991.

Coogan, Tim Pat, *Michael Collins: The Man Who Made Ireland.* Boulder, CO, 1996; originally published 1992.

Cowling, Maurice, *The Impact of Labour, 1920–1924: The Beginning of Modern British Politics.* London, 1971.

Cronin, Mike, ed., *The Failure of British Fascism: The Far Right and the Fight for Political Recognition.* London, 1996.

Dean, Carolyn J., *The Self and Its Pleasures: Bataille, Lacan, and the History of the Decentered Subject.* Ithaca, NY, 1992.

Dummett, Ann and Andrew Nicol, *Subjects, Citizens, Aliens and Others: Nationality and Immigration Law.* London, 1990.

Echewa, T. Obinkaram, *I Saw the Sky Catch Fire.* New York, 1992.

Edkins, Jenny, "Remembering Relationality: Trauma Time and Politics," in Duncan Bell, ed., *Memory, Trauma and World Politics: Reflections on the Relationship Between Past and Present.* London, 2006.

Erikson, Kai, "Notes on Trauma and Community," in Cathy Caruth, ed., *Trauma: Explorations in Memory.* Baltimore, 1995.

Farr, Barbara Storm, *The Development and Impact of Right-Wing-Politics in Britain, 1903–1932.* 1987.

Figley, Charles R. and Rolf J. Kleber, "Beyond the 'Victim': Secondary Traumatic Stress," in Rolf J. Kleber, Charles R. Figley, and Berthold P.R. Gersons, eds, *Beyond Trauma: Cultural and Society Dynamics.* New York, 1995.

Flory, Harriette, "William Joynson-Hicks, Lord Brentford: A Political Biography," unpublished dissertation, University of Cincinnati, 1975.

Foster, Hal, "Armour Fou," *October*, 56 (Spring 1991), 64–97.

——, "Postmodernism in Parallax," *October*, 63 (Winter 1993), 3–20.

Furneaux, Rupert, *Massacre at Amritsar.* London, 1963.

Fussell, Paul, *The Great War and Modern Memory.* New York, 1975.

Gailey, Harry A., *The Road to Aba: A Study of British Administrative Policy in Eastern Nigeria.* New York, 1970.

Gilbert, Martin, *Churchill, A Life.* New York, 1991.

Gottlieb, Julie V., *Feminine Fascism: Women in Britain's Fascist Movement, 1923–1945.* London, 2000.

—— and Thomas P. Linehan, eds, *The Culture of Fascism: Visions of the Far Right in Britain.* London, 2004.

Graves, Charles, *Invasion By Virus. Can It Happen Again?* London, 1969.

Grayzel, Susan R., *Women's Identities at War: Gender, Motherhood, and Politics in Britain and France during the First World War.* Chapel Hill, NC, 1999.

Green, E.H., *Ideologies of Conservatism: Conservative Political Ideas in the Twentieth Century.* Oxford, 2002.

Gregory, Adrian, *The Silence of Memory: Armistice Day, 1919–1946*. Oxford, 1994.

Herman, Judith Lewis, *Trauma and Recovery: The Aftermath of Violence—From Domestic Abuse to Political Terror*. New York, 1992.

Hynes, Samuel, *A War Imagined: The First World War and British Culture*. New York, 1992.

Jarvis, David, "The Shaping of Conservative Electoral Hegemony, 1918–1939," in Jon Lawrence and Miles Taylor, eds, *Party, State and Society: Electoral Behaviour in Britain since 1920*. Aldershot, 1997.

Jenkinson, Jacqueline, "The 1919 Race Riots in Britain: Their Background and Consequences," unpublished thesis, University of Edinburgh, 1987.

Joynson-Hicks, Sir William, *Communist Plotting: Lessons from the General Strike*. 1926.

Judd, Allen, *Ford Madox Ford*. Cambridge, Ma., 1990.

Kent, Susan Kingsley, *Gender and Power in Britain, 1640–1990*. London, 1999.

——, *Making Peace: The Reconstruction of Gender in Interwar Britain*. Princeton, 1993.

——, *Sex and Suffrage in Britain, 1860–1914*. Princeton, 1987.

Kushner, Tony, "The Paradox of Prejudice: The Impact of Organised Antisemitism in Britain during an Anti-Nazi War", in Tony Kushner and Kenneth Lunn, eds, *Traditions of Intolerance: Historical Perspectives on Fascism and Race Discourse in Britain*. Manchester, 1989.

Kushner, Tony and Kenneth Lund, eds, *Traditions of Intolerance: Historical Perspectives on Fascism and Race Discourse in Britain*. Manchester, 1989.

Laqueur, Thomas W., "Memory and Naming in the Great War," in John R. Gillis, ed., *Commemorations: The Politics of National Identity*. Princeton, 1994.

Laub, Dori, "Truth and Testimony: The Process and the Struggle," in Cathy Caruth, ed., *Trauma: Explorations in Memory*. Baltimore, 1995.

Lawrence, Jon, "Forging a Peaceable Kingdom: War, Violence, and Fear of Brutalization in Post-First World War Britain," *Journal of Modern History*, 75 (September 2003), 557–589.

Laybourn, Keith, *The General Strike of 1926*. Manchester, 1993.

Leese, Peter, *Shell Shock: Traumatic Neurosis and the British Soldiers of the First World War*. New York, 2002.

Light, Alison, *Forever England: Femininity, Literature and Conservatism Between the Wars*. London, 1991.

Lunn, Kenneth, "The Ideology and Impact of the British Fascists in the 1920s," in Kushner, Tony and Kenneth Lund, eds, *Traditions of Intolerance: Historical Perspectives on Fascism and Race Discourse in Britain*. Manchester, 1989.

Maguire, Richard Charles, " 'The Fascists . . . are . . . to be depended upon.' The British Government, Fascists and Strike-breaking during 1925 and 1926," in Nigel Copsey and David Renton, eds, *British Fascism, the Labour Movement and the State*. Basingstoke, 2005.

Mandler, Peter, *The English National Character: The History of an Idea from Edmund Burke to Tony Blair*. New Haven, 2006.

Macardle, Dorothy, *The Irish Republic, A Documented Chronicle of the Anglo-Irish Conflict and the Partitioning of Ireland, with a Detailed Account of the Period 1916–1923*. Dublin, 1999; originally published 1937.

McCarthy, Helen, "Parties, Voluntary Associations, and Democratic Politics in Interwar Britain," *The Historical Journal*, 50, 4 (2007), 891–912.

McKibbin, Ross, *The Ideologies of Class: Social Relations in Britain, 1880–1950*. Oxford, 1994.

Melman, Billie, ed., *Borderlines: Genders and Identities in War and Peace, 1870–1930*. New York, 1998.

——, *Women and the Popular Imagination in the Twenties: Flappers and Nymphs*. New York, 1988.

Middlemas, Keith and John Barnes, *Baldwin, A Biography*. London, 1969.

Moorhouse, Geoffrey, *Hell's Foundations: A Social History of the Town of Bury in the Aftermath of the Gallipoli Campaign*. New York, 1992.

Morgan, Kenneth O., *Consensus and Disunity. The Lloyd George Coalition Government, 1918–1922*. Oxford, 1979.

Mowat, Charles Loch, *Britain Between the Wars, 1918–1940*. Chicago, 1955.

Neligan, David, *The Spy in the Castle*. London, 1999; originally published 1968.

Panayi, Panikos, *The Enemy in Our Midst: Germans in Britain During the First World War*. New York, 1991.

——, "Introduction," in Panikos Panayi, ed., *Racial Violence in Britain, 1840–1950*. Leicester, 1993.

Pedersen, Susan, "From National Crisis to 'National Crisis:' British Politics, 1914–1931," *Journal of British Studies*, 33, 3 (July 1994), 322–335.

Peele, Gillian and Chris Cook, eds, *The Politics of Reappraisal, 1918–1939*. New York, 1975.

Perkins, Anne, *A Very British Strike: 3 May–12 May 1926*. London, 2006.

Ray, Larry, "Mourning, Melancholia and Violence," in Duncan Bell., ed., *Memory, Trauma and World Politics: Reflections on the Relationship Between Past and Present*. London, 2006.

Reinders, Robert, "Racialism on the Left. E.D. Morel and the 'Black Horror on the Rhine," *International Review of Social History*, 13 (1968), 1–28.

Renshaw, Patrick, *The General Strike*. London, 1975.

Rich, Paul, B., *Race and Empire in British Politics*. Cambridge, 1986.

Rosaldo, Renato, "Grief and a Headhunter's Rage: On the Cultural Force of Emotions," in Edward M. Bruner, ed., *Text, Play, and Story: The Construction and Reconstruction of Self and Society*. Washington, D.C, 1984.

Rose, Jonathan, *The Edwardian Temperament, 1895–1919*. Athens, OH, 1986.

Santner, Eric L., *Stranded Objects: Mourning, Memory, and Film in Postwar Germany*. Ithaca, NY, 1990.

Sayer, Derek, "British Reaction to the Amritsar Massacre, 1919–1920," *Past and Present*, 131 (1991), 130–164.

Schivelbusch, Wolfgang, *The Railway Journey: The Industrialization of Time and Space in the 19th Century*. Berkeley, 1977.

Smelser, Neil J., "Psychological Trauma and Cultural Trauma," in Jeffrey C. Alexander, Ron Eyerman, Bernhard, Giesen, Neil J. Smelser, and Piotr Sztompka, eds, *Cultural Trauma and Collective Identity*. Berkeley, 2004.

Smith, Harold L., ed., *British Feminism in the Twentieth Century*. Aldershot, 1990.

Spurling, Hilary, *Ivy: The Life of I. Compton-Burnett*. New York, 1984.

Squire, Larry R. and Eric R. Kandel, *Memory from Mind to Molecules*. New York, 1999.

Stevenson, J., "Conservatism and the Future of Fascism in Interwar Britain," in M. Blinkhorn, ed., *Fascists and Conservatives*. London, 1990.

Stone, Dan, *Breeding Superman: Nietzsche, Race and Eugenics in Edwardian and Interwar Britain.* Liverpool, 2002.

Stone, Martin, "Shellshock and the Psychologists," in W.F. Bynum, Roy Porter, and Michael Shepherd, eds, *The Anatomy of Madness: Essays in the History of Psychiatry. Volume II: Institutions and Society.* London, 1985.

Symons, Julian, *The General Strike: A Historical Portrait.* London, 1957.

Tabili, Laura, *"We Ask for British Justice," Workers and Racial Difference in Later Imperial Britain.* Ithaca, NY, 1994.

Tate, Trudi, *Modernism, History and the First World War.* Manchester, 1998.

Theweleit, Klaus, *Male Fantasies, Volume I: Women, Floods, Bodies, History.* Minneapolis, 1987; originally published, 1977.

Townshend, Charles, *Political Violence in Ireland: Government and Resistance since 1848.* Oxford, 1983.

Turner, John, *British Politics and the Great War, Coalition and Conflict, 1915–1918.* New Haven, 1992.

Van Allen, Judith, " 'Sitting On a Man:' Colonization and the Lost Political Institutions of Igbo Women," in Sharon W. Tiffany, ed., *Women and Society: An Anthropological Reader.* St. Albans, VT, 1979.

Van der Kolk, Bessel and Onno Van der Hart, "The Intrusive Past: The Flexibility of Memory and the Engraving of Trauma," in Cathy Caruth, ed., *Trauma: Explorations in Memory.* Baltimore, 1995.

Watson, Janet K., *Fighting Different Wars: Experience, Memory, and the First World War in Britain.* New York, 2004.

Webber, G.C., *The Ideology of the British Right, 1918–1939.* London, 1986.

Williamson, Philip, "The Doctrinal Politics of Stanley Baldwin," in Michael Bentley, ed., *Public and Private Doctrine: Essays in British History presented to Maurice Cowling.* Cambridge, 1993.

——, *National Crisis and National Government: British Politics, the Economy and Empire, 1926–1932.* Cambridge, 1992.

Wilson, Trevor, *The Myriad Faces of War: Britain and the Great War, 1914–1918.* Cambridge, 1986.

Winter, Jay, *The Great War and the British People.* Cambridge, Ma., 1986.

——, "Shell-Shock and the Cultural History of the Great War," *Journal of Contemporary History*, 35, 1 (2000), 7–11.

——, *Sites of Memory, Sites of Mourning: The Great War in European Cultural History.* Cambridge, 1995.

—— and Antoine Prost, *The Great War in History: Debates and Controversies, 1914 to the Present.* Cambridge, 2005.

Woollacott, Angela, *On Her Their Lives Depend: Munitions Workers in the Great War.* Berkeley, 1994.

Young, Alan, *The Harmony of Illusions: Inventing Post-Traumatic Stress Disorder.* Princeton, NJ, 1995.

Index

Aba Commission, 176, 177, 178
Aba riots, 163–78
Ackerly, J.R., 29
Africans, 9, 45, 57, 63
African World, 174
air raids, 2, 14, 15, 17, 61
Aldington, Richard, 7, 13, 30, 31, 116, 124
Alec-Tweedie, Mrs, 38, 39
Alexander, Jeffrey, 25
Alford, C. Fred, 28
aliens, 4, 5, 9, 41–5, 48, 51, 54, 58, 61–3, 119, 127, 131, 146
Aliens Order, 45, 54
Aliens' Restriction Act
    of 1905, 44
    of 1914, 41, 44, 45
    of 1919, 5, 40, 41, 51, 54, 58, 60, 62
Ampthill, Lord, 75, 76, 82, 88
Amritsar massacre, 5, 64–77, 80, 85, 86, 89
Anderson, Sir John, 95, 103
Anglo-Indians, 66, 71, 72, 73, 77, 79, 80, 87
annihilation, 6, 9, 11, 57, 58, 80, 115, 155, 160, 161, 165, 170, 190, 193
anti-Semitism, 43, 60, 61
Anti-Waste League, 125
anxiety, 13, 17, 18, 37, 38, 101, 133, 153, 169
Arabs, 45, 181
Archer, Thomas, 47
Armistice, 1, 8, 14, 18, 24, 32, 42, 111, 120, 125
artillery, 2, 12, 13, 25, 92
    see also shelling
Armistice Day, 32
Asians, 45, 83
Asquith, Herbert H., 37, 87, 117, 133
Auxiliaries, 34, 97, 98, 108, 111
    see also Black and Tans

Balbriggan, 96, 118
Bernard, Lieutenant-Colonel D.K., 102
Bevin, Ernest, 185
Billing, Noel Pemberton, 40, 42, 43, 44
Bingham, Adrian, 160, 161
Birkenhead, Lord, 86, 88, 128, 129
birth control, 150, 157
Black and Tans, 34, 72, 91, 94–103, 106, 108, 109, 111–15, 117, 118, 121, 138
    see also Auxiliaries
Black Friday, 124
"blacks", 5, 33, 45, 46–9, 51–9
Blackwood's Magazine, 76
black troops, 5, 40, 55, 56, 57, 203
Boards of Guardians Act, 141
Board of Trade, 52, 53
bolsheviks, 9, 42, 51, 57, 58, 60, 85, 87, 120, 125, 126, 128, 129, 155
Bondfield, Margaret, 152
Bottomley, Horatio, 41
"Britain for the British", 41, 43, 45
British Broadcasting Corporation (BBC), 123, 187
British empire, 7, 8, 9, 51, 86, 87, 88, 120, 121, 159, 161, 177, 189
British Fascists, 60, 62, 131
British Gazette, 133, 135–7
British Medical Journal, 22
British Union of Fascists, 59, 193
British Worker, 139, 140
Brittain, Vera, 7, 18, 19, 29, 32
Burgess, Anthony, 23, 24, 28
Burgoyne, Lieutenant-Colonel Sir Alan, 130
Bush, Barbara, 55
Bushaway, Bob, 32

Caine, Sir Hall, 146
Calvin, W.H., 25
Cardiff, 45, 47, 48, 55, 61, 62, 135, 152
Cardiff Watch Committee, 48

Carlin, Thomas, 45
Carson, Sir Edward, 41, 75, 81, 82, 88, 91
Caruth, Cathy, 25
Carver, Christian, 13
Catholicism, 9, 78, 114
Chamberlain, Austen, 83, 125
Chamberlain, Neville, 124, 131, 141, 188, 193
Chapin, Harold, 13
Chapman, Guy, 14, 30
Chelmsford, Lord, 65, 72, 73, 82–4
Chesterton, G.K., 118
Chinese, 46, 47, 50, 189
Churchill, Winston, 85, 87, 94, 95, 102, 103, 104, 107, 108, 111, 119, 120, 126, 129, 131–3, 137, 142, 161, 182, 183, 189, 194
Civil Constabulary Reserve, 136
Clynes, J.R., 185
Coalition government, 37, 40, 80, 83, 125, 126, 142
coal subsidy, 131
Cockerill, Brigadier-General George, 158, 160
collective psyche, 5, 6, 9, 91, 195
  see also national psyche
Collett, Nigel, 67, 73, 74, 78, 79
Colonial Office, 52, 53, 54, 170, 174, 181
Coloured Alien Seamen Order, 54
Comaroff, Jean, 10
Compton-Burnett, Ivy, 14, 18, 23
Congress party, 70, 71, 182
consciousness, 7, 10, 11, 24, 27, 72, 113, 126
conservatism, 3, 4, 32, 40, 41, 63
Conservative party, 4, 5, 62, 63, 125, 127, 128, 130, 157, 182, 193
Contemporary Review, 57, 142
Coogan, Tim, 96, 102
Cork, 95, 98, 102, 106, 107, 117
coupon election, 40
Cowar, Duncan, 45
Crawford, James Edward, 167
crawling order, 71, 72, 78, 86
Croft, Henry Page, 40, 42, 60, 82
Curzon, Lord, 86

Dáil Éireann, 93
Daily Express, 21, 22, 32, 125, 127, 135, 153, 156, 162, 163, 189, 193, 194
Daily Herald, 49, 50, 55, 56, 117, 139–41, 173, 191, 192, 194
Daily Mail, 40, 41, 74, 125, 128, 129, 134, 135, 136, 140, 143, 147, 149, 150, 152–6, 160–3, 170–3, 182, 189, 190, 193
Daily News, 99, 117, 151, 170
Daily Telegraph, 78, 105, 173
Daily Worker, 173, 176
Davidson, J.C.C., 130, 131, 135, 138, 193
Dawson, W.H., 57
Defence of India Act, 65
Defense of the Realm Act (DORA), 18, 38
Delhi, 65, 77, 82
demobilization, 30, 31, 35–7, 48, 94
democracy, 4, 7, 8, 81, 85, 157, 189, 192, 194
Dexter, Mary, 20
Die-Hards, 4, 5, 60, 61
Dillon, John, 92
dismemberment, 13, 17, 24
dissociation, 22, 25, 27
divided self, 10, 11, 27
domesticity, 8, 153
Doolittle, Hilda (HD), 2, 18
Doyle, Arthur Conan, 38
Dry, Thomas, 13
Dublin, 81, 90, 92, 93, 95, 97, 103, 109, 117
Duckworth, Henry, 137
Duff, Duncan, 96, 97, 103, 112, 113, 115, 116
Dyer, Brigadier-General Reginald, 71–91, 107–9

East End News, 46
Eastern Post and City Chronicle, 146
Easter Rising, 33, 92, 114
Edwardians, 11, 27
Edward VIII, 194
Egypt, 13, 88, 89, 124, 181
Eight Hours Act, 142
Eligibility of Women Act, 150

Ellis, Havelock, 11
emasculation, 153, 155, 159
Emergency Powers Act, 131
enfranchisement of women, 5, 33, 37, 148–52, 154–7, 159–63, 193
see also women's suffrage
Englishness, 4, 7, 8, 9, 34
Evening Standard, 146

Fabian Women's Group, 55
Factory Times, 151
fascism/fascists, 3, 6, 9, 31, 40, 59, 60, 62, 63, 161, 192–4
Federation of Women Teachers, 55
feminism, 2, 150, 156
Fennel, Dr. Rufus, 48
Finlay, Lord, 75, 76, 78, 81, 82
Fisher, H.A.L., 111
Fitzpatrick, Sir Percy, 32
flappers, 39, 153–6, 163, 179
flashbacks, 28, 29
Ford, Ford Madox, 1, 13
Forster, E.M., 11
fragmentation, 3, 6, 12, 27, 28, 30, 160, 165
freicorps, 58, 59
French, 55, 56, 57, 112
Freud, Sigmund, 27, 32
Fussell, Paul, 32

Galloway, John, 30
Gandhi, Mohandas, 65, 66, 77, 83, 182
Garvin, J.L., 183, 184, 187, 188
gender, 20, 28, 31, 38–40, 53, 153, 163
General Strike, 4, 5, 122, 123, 126, 133, 141–3, 147, 161, 190
Germans, 6, 12, 21, 31, 40, 41, 55, 57, 85, 92, 101, 132
Germany, 5, 6, 31, 35, 38, 56, 57, 85, 131, 181, 187, 190, 193, 194
Gibbs, Philip, 2, 14, 17, 31, 35, 36, 111, 117, 119, 120, 151, 190
Glasgow, 45, 46, 49, 89, 123, 124, 136, 138
Graves, Robert, 7, 29

Great War, 1, 2, 6–12, 25, 33, 35, 36, 60, 64, 85, 92, 95, 112–14, 126, 132, 133, 137, 140, 141, 153, 160, 180, 182, 183, 186, 187, 190, 195
see also World War I
Green, E.H.H., 126
Green, Margaret, 166
Greenwood, Sir Hamar, 88, 95, 96, 98, 100, 103, 105, 108, 110, 114, 119, 120
Gregory, Adrian, 19, 32
Gregory, Lady Augusta, 99, 100–2, 112
grief, 3, 14, 16, 18, 19, 25, 26, 28, 32, 195
guerilla warfare, 113, 117
Guest, Haden, 138

Hall, Lieutenant-Colonel Sir F., 158
hallucination, 1, 21, 22, 24, 29
Harlen, Michael, 156
Hassan, Abdulia, 46
Haynes, E.S.P., 13
Henderson, Arthur, 181, 185
Herman, Judith, 24, 25, 33
Hill, Lieutenant Richard, 168, 172
Hitler, Adolf, 161
Holliday, G., 22
home front, 2, 20
Home Office, 41, 50, 53–5, 62, 130, 131
Home Rule, Irish, 91–3
Home Secretary, 41, 42, 44, 54, 62, 127, 149
House of Commons, 5, 41, 65, 73, 75, 81, 82, 83, 87, 100, 105, 130, 131, 138, 139, 144, 157, 162, 192
House of Lords, 73, 81, 86, 88, 159
Hunter Commission, 71, 72, 74, 78, 82, 85
Hunter-Weston, Lieutenant-General Sir Aylmer, 86
Hyde Park, 48, 134
hysteria, 20, 23, 61, 154, 165

Igbo Women's War, 5, 164–79
Illustrated London News, 21
India, 60, 64, 65, 69, 72, 73, 75–83, 85–90, 108, 120, 138, 156, 159, 169, 181, 182

Indian Civil Service (ICS), 65, 79
Indian Mutiny of 1857, 77, 79, 80
Indians, 45, 50, 63, 65, 66, 67, 70, 71,
   72, 74, 79, 82, 85, 91
India Office, 53
influenza epidemic (flu), 14, 15, 20–3,
   27, 32, 65
Ireland, 33, 34, 60, 72, 88–95, 97,
   103–5, 108–10, 112, 113,
   115–18, 120, 121, 124, 136, 138,
   156, 169
Irish, 5, 9, 14, 33, 59, 63, 88, 89, 91–4,
   97, 103, 108, 110, 111, 114–17,
   119, 121, 138
Irish Republican Army (IRA), 93–5, 97,
   102–4, 106–8, 111, 115, 124
Irish Situation Committee, 110, 116,
   119, 120
Irish Volunteers, 92, 93
Irving, Deputy Commissioner Miles,
   66–8, 72
Italy, 31, 182, 193

Jallianwallah Bagh, 64, 65, 68–70,
   73–7, 80, 85, 91
Jamaican, 47
Jameson, Storm, 18
Jeudwine, Lieutenant-General Hugh,
   104
Jews, 4, 5, 9, 33, 42–4, 51, 54, 58–63,
   83–5, 181
John Bull, 40
Johnson, Tom, 45
Jones, Kennedy, 40
Jones, Thomas, 95, 103
Joynson-Hicks, William, 40, 42, 43,
   54, 60, 62, 76, 127, 129–31, 133,
   135–7, 139, 147, 149, 150, 157

Keeling, Frederic, 13
Kenealy, Reverend, A.E.J., 78, 79
Keynes, J.M., 183
Kindersley, Major G.M., 169
Kitchin, A.J.W., 66, 67
Kushner, Tony, 59

Labour Commission, 112, 118, 121
Labour party, 2, 3, 4, 5, 37, 41, 42, 60,
   61, 81, 87, 117, 120, 123–31, 138,
   140, 142, 143, 146–8, 150, 152,
   155, 157, 160–3, 180–9, 191–5
Lacan, Jacques, 27, 28
Lancashire Fusiliers, 29
Lancet, 19, 21–3
Lansbury, George, 140, 141, 142, 185,
   192
Laski, Harold, 187
Law, Andrew Bonar, 5, 37, 40, 91
Lawrence, Susan, 152
Leeds Mercury, 151
Liberal party, 3, 8, 37, 41, 81, 83, 84,
   117, 118, 123, 125–7, 132, 180,
   183–5, 187
Liverpool, 16, 44, 45, 47, 48, 50,
   52, 54
Liverpool Courier, 48, 51
Lloyd George, David, 37, 40, 57, 83,
   86, 95, 103, 105, 108, 111, 115,
   124–6, 161, 182–4
London, 2, 14, 16, 22, 43–6, 50, 61,
   81, 122–4, 132, 133, 135, 136,
   138, 141, 156, 162, 165, 174,
   180–2
London Naval Conference, 181
Long, Walter, 116
lost generation, 10
Lugard, Sir Frederick D., 57, 58

Macaulay, Rose, 27
MacCurtain, Thomas, 95
MacDonald, Ramsay, 42, 126–30, 134,
   142, 161–3, 181–4, 186–8
Macready, General Neville, 88, 94, 95,
   100, 102, 105–10, 115, 119–21,
   136
McKibbin, Ross, 62, 126
Magner, Canon, 96, 98, 115
Manchester Guardian, 90, 117, 142,
   147, 161–3, 170, 173, 191
Mandler, Peter, 8
Manning, Frederic, 13
Mansfield, Katherine, 19
marriage, 37, 127, 157
martial law, 71, 72, 92, 106, 108–10,
   115, 120
Martin, Kingsley, 194
Marx, Karl, 10
Mason, William, 13

massacre, 65, 70–3, 75, 80, 85, 87, 107, 155, 173, 176, 193
Massingham, H.J., 118
Masterson, C.F.G., 142, 145
Matrimonial Causes Act, 150
Maxwell, W.N., 1
melancholia, 32
memory, 2, 3, 13, 14, 24, 25, 29, 32, 39, 78, 164
Mesopotamia, 120
MI5, 136
Middle-Class Union, 125
miners, 60, 90, 111, 122–4, 129, 140–2
Ministry of Health, 20, 22
Ministry of Labour, 48, 52, 53
miscegenation, 50, 51, 53, 55, 57–9
Monmouth Evening Post, 47
Montagu-Chelmsford reforms, 65, 181
Montague, C.E., 28, 65, 72, 81–85
Morel, E.D., 55, 56
Morning Post, 4, 40, 51, 60, 73, 75, 76, 77, 78, 82, 83, 84, 88, 117, 133, 173, 175
Morris, Richard, 140
Mosley, Sir Oswald, 59, 161, 183, 186, 194
motherhood, 37, 153
mourning, 4, 14, 19, 32
Muslims, 46, 66
Mussolini, Benito, 161, 181, 192
mutilation, 95, 101

Narayan, Pandit Jagat, 85
nation, 2, 4, 5, 7–9, 14, 15, 20, 32, 33, 38, 40, 42, 44, 51, 57, 59, 63–5, 83, 86, 88, 89, 91, 118, 119, 122, 128–30, 132–4, 136, 138–40, 142–8, 154, 156, 157, 179, 180, 183, 185–9
national character, 8, 43
National Citizens' Union, 62
"national crisis", 180, 182, 184, 185, 187–90, 192, 195
National Federation of Women's Workers, 55
National government, 5, 52, 182, 184–95
national identity, 33, 34, 63, 195
national psyche, 6, 91, 195

National Review, 4, 40, 60, 117, 163
National Sailor's and Firemen's Union, 49
National Union of Societies for Equal Citizenship, 55, 79, 173
Nation and Athenaeum, 143, 146, 148
Newman, Sir George, 20
New York, 113, 180, 191
Nield, Sir H., 43
Nigeria, 57, 163–5, 170–9, 181

O'Dwyer, Sir Michael, 65, 67, 72, 78, 79
Oloko, 164

pacifists, 40, 133
Palestine, 181
Pankhurst, Sylvia, 15
patriotism, 4, 128, 140, 144, 161, 188, 189, 191
Peachey, Bert, 30
Perkins, Anne, 128, 135, 138
Pettigrew, Eileen, 22
Pitt, Bernard, 12
Playne, Caroline, 2, 15, 17, 19, 22
Poland, 61, 124
police, 31, 35, 45–9, 52, 54, 68, 70, 72, 73, 88, 93–6, 103–11, 114–17, 121, 124, 131, 134–9, 146, 165, 171, 172, 175, 176, 191
politics, 3, 37, 40, 59, 125, 126, 148, 156, 183–6, 190
Porter, Katherine Anne, 23
Price, Morgan Philips, 193
Protestant, 91, 99, 119
Prussianism, 7, 8, 85
post-traumatic stress disorder (PTSD), 2, 4, 15, 34, 72, 91, 94–103, 106, 108, 109, 111–15, 117, 118, 121, 138
  see also trauma, war neuroses
Punch, 153
Punjab, 60, 65–70, 74, 76, 78, 79, 85, 89

Quinn, Ellen, 96, 102
Quinn, Malachi, 99
Quit India movement, 64

race, 8, 9, 35, 43, 51, 53–60, 81, 82, 84, 119, 139, 146, 147, 154, 157, 182, 188
race riots, 5, 31, 34, 40, 45–53, 59
rape, 77, 79, 80, 95, 100, 101
Rathbone, Eleanor, 55
Rathbone, Irene, 17, 28–30, 35, 39
Ray, Larry, 32, 179
Read, Herbert, 30, 116
Red Cross, 12
Redmond, John, 92
religion, 10, 11, 63
repatriation, 45, 52, 53
Representation of the People Act of 1918, 37, 149
reprisals, 5, 72, 88, 91, 94–99, 102–128, 138
Rhondda, Lady, 49, 118
Rowlatt Acts, 65, 66
Royal Army Medical Corps, 13
Royal Irish Constabulary (RIC), 93–5, 97, 103–5, 108, 113, 121
Russia, 42, 62, 123, 124, 126–8
Russian revolution, 37, 42, 123

sacrifice, 7, 8, 30, 37, 48, 85, 115, 140, 146, 185, 188, 190
Saklatvala, Shapurji, 127
Salisbury, Lord Robert, 5
Samuel, Herbert, 141, 184
Samuel, Samuel, 158, 159
Sassoon, Siegfried, 7, 16, 32, 38, 118
Sayers, Dorothy, 26
Scott, James, 29
separate spheres, 40, 151
Setalvad, Sir C.H., 85
Sex Disqualification Removal Act, 150
sexual attacks, 36, 56, 101
sexual disorders, 40, 43, 155
sexuality, 28, 36–40, 42, 44, 50, 56–8, 153, 155, 160, 163, 165–9
sex war, 159
shattering, 6, 7, 12, 26, 28, 126
shell shock, 1, 2, 3, 5, 6, 10–12, 15, 24
    see also trauma, war neuroses
shelling, 12, 13, 15
    see also artillery
Sherwood, Marcella, 66, 71, 78, 79
Sierra Leone, 45

Simon Commission, 182
Simon, Sir John, 132, 133, 145–7, 181
Simpson, Wallis, 194
Sinn Féin, 93, 96, 99, 102, 103, 110, 114, 115, 117
Smith, A. Burnett, 16, 18
Snowden, Philip, 187
socialism, 4, 8, 40, 58, 62, 120, 123, 125–9, 145, 150, 155, 156, 160, 161, 163, 185, 187, 190, 193, 194
Somme, 18
South Wales Evening Express, 48, 49
Spectator, 4, 40, 75, 117, 174
Spoor, Ben, 87
Stopes, Marie, 150
Sturgis, Mark, 103, 105
subjectivity, 5, 10, 11, 80, 165
suicide, 18, 23, 29
Sunday Times, 104
Symons, Julian, 123

terrorism, 81, 85, 86, 98, 104, 141
Thirsk and Malton Conservative Association, 131
Thomas, J.H., 138, 187
Thompson, Graeme, 170
The Times, 22, 38, 50, 60, 61, 66, 84, 99, 105, 117, 118, 127, 133, 134, 136, 144, 145, 161–3, 170–3, 175, 190
Time and Tide, 36
Tomb of the Unknowns, 32
torture, 1, 71, 72, 80, 92
Trades Union Congress (TUC), 55, 122, 123, 126, 131, 134, 139, 141, 142, 185–157
trauma, 2, 3, 4, 5, 6, 7, 9, 10–12, 15, 20, 24, 25, 27, 28, 31, 33, 64, 65, 73, 91, 112, 113, 115, 118, 178, 179, 182, 186, 193, 195
    see also post-traumatic stress disorder (PTSD); shell shock
trade union movement, 139, 142
Trades Disputes Act of 1927, 142
trenches, 12, 13, 15, 16, 20, 21, 25, 30, 153
Trevelyan, Charles, 193
Triple Alliance, 124

Tudor, Major-General Henry, 94, 95, 102, 103, 106, 107, 109
Twickenham Conservative Association, 147

Ukraine, 61
unemployment insurance, 125, 181, 184, 185
"un-Englishness", 4, 82, 119, 147
Union of Democratic Control, 55, 56

venereal disease, 36–7, 38
vengeance, 33, 53, 77, 79, 96
Verdun, 30
veterans, 15, 22, 28–31, 35, 112, 113
Viceroy of India, 65, 181
Victorians, 10, 80
violence, 4, 5, 6, 9, 20, 26, 28, 31, 34, 35, 36, 45, 46, 48, 50, 55, 59, 66, 68, 71, 72, 74, 78, 86, 91, 95, 101, 103, 106, 108, 111–13, 115, 117, 118, 135, 136, 138, 139, 147, 156, 159, 163, 168
Voluntary Aid Detachments (VAD), 15, 17
von Arnim, Elizabeth, 27

Wakefield, C.C., 145
War Graves Commission, 32
war neuroses, 2, 19, 20, 22
    see also trauma, shell shock
Warner, Sir Courtenay, 42
war novels, 2, 7, 13, 17, 26, 27, 31
War Office, 54, 136
Wathen, Gerard, wife of, 67
Watson, Angus, 146
Watson, Sir Francis, 155
Webb, Beatrice, 11, 136, 185, 186, 193
Webber, G.C., 63
Wedgwood, Colonel, 41–2
Weekly Summary, 103, 104, 105, 114, 115

Welsh, 14, 42, 119
West Hartlepool, 15
West Indians, 9, 45, 50, 63
Westminster Gazette, 117
West, Rebecca, 26
West, Samuel, 22
Wild, Sir Ernest, 41
Wilkinson, Ellen, 152
Williamson, Philip, 183, 186, 192
Williams, Ralph, 50
Wilson, Sir Henry, 79, 95, 98, 102, 103, 105–9, 115, 119–21, 124
Wilson, Theodore, 13
Wimsey, Lord Peter, 26
Winter, Jay, 2, 3
Winterbourne, George, 13
Woman's Leader, 55, 57, 79, 173
Women's Auxiliary Army Corps (WAAC), 17, 38
Women's Cooperative Guild, 55
Women's International League for Peace and Freedom, 55, 56
women's suffrage:
    see also enfranchisement of women, 3, 4, 7, 37, 79, 149–51, 155, 158–60, 162, 163, 178
Woods, Margaret, 137
Woolf, Virginia, 118, 122, 123, 135, 141
Wooten, Charles, 47
working class, 3, 4, 8, 9, 58, 119, 123, 125, 126, 136, 143, 148, 152, 156, 191
World War 1
    see also, Great War, 12, 15, 188
Worthington-Evans, Lamington, 124

Zeppelin raids, 16, 132
Zinoviev, Grigory, 128, 155
Zinoviev letter, 61, 128

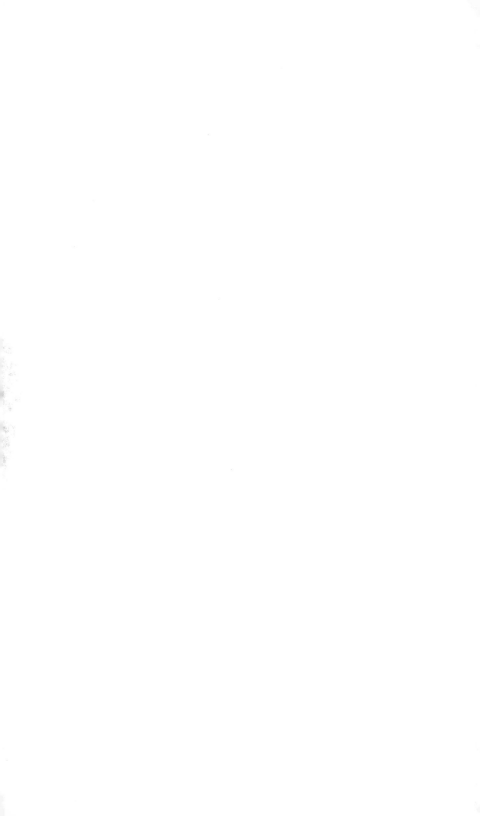

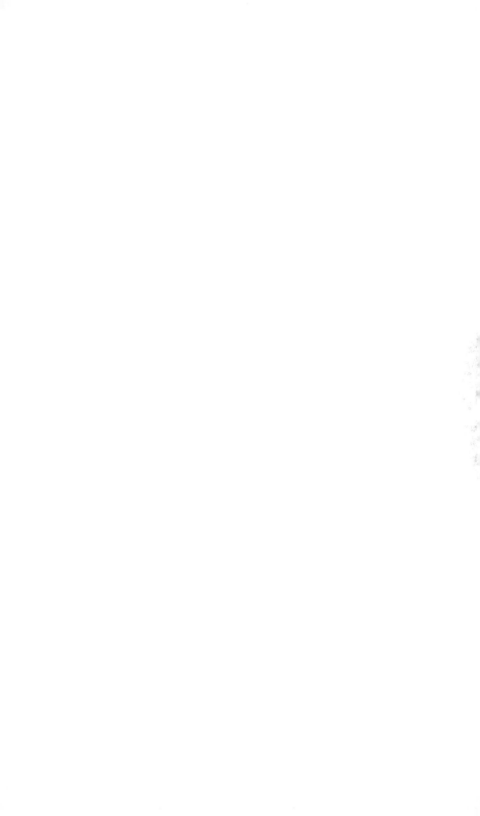